Manage High Bl Pressure with Healthy Diet

Easy, Delicious and Nutritious Recipes

BY: SOPHIA FREEMAN

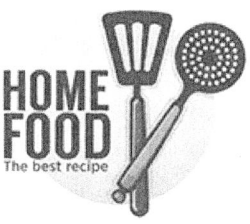

© 2020 Sophia Freeman All Rights Reserved

COPYRIGHTED

Liability

This publication is meant as an informational tool. The individual purchaser accepts all liability if damages occur because of following the directions or guidelines set out in this publication. The Author bears no responsibility for reparations caused by the misuse or misinterpretation of the content.

Copyright

The content of this publication is solely for entertainment purposes and is meant to be purchased by one individual. Permission is not given to any individual who copies, sells or distributes parts or the whole of this publication unless it is explicitly given by the Author in writing.

Table of Contents

Introduction 7

   Scallop Salad 9

   Salmon Satay 12

   Salmon Tostadas 16

   Sirloin Salad 19

   Zucchini Noodles with Pesto 22

   Pistachio Crusted Mahi Mahi 25

   Creamy Tomato Soup 29

   Pesto Penne with Chicken Veggies 31

   Lettuce Wraps 34

   Shrimp with Artichoke Salad 37

   Turkey Burger 40

   Baked Chicken Asparagus 43

   Baked Tuna Steak 46

   Sweet Potatoes Stuffed with Chicken Curry 49

   Roasted Mushrooms 52

Seared Tuna with Salad 55

Shrimp Pesto 58

Provençal Fish Fillets 61

Crunchy Salmon Fillet 64

Pot Roast 67

Curry Fish 70

Salmon Salad 73

Garlic Shrimp with Spinach 76

Salmon with Kale Creamy Dressing 79

Herbed Scallops with Asparagus 82

Zucchini Noodles with Meat Veggies 85

Turkey Salad 88

Rosemary Turkey Roast 91

Spaghetti Squash with Tomato Basil 94

Mushroom Wrap 97

Chicken Salad with Avocado Pineapple 100

Beef Burgundy with Mashed Potatoes 103

Tofu Soup with Veggies 107

Jerk Chicken 110

Steak with Mushroom Sauce 113

Chicken Pasta Primavera 116

Lemon Chicken 119

Citrus Salmon Grilled Veggies 122

Beef Kebab 125

Grilled Veggies 129

Garlic Fish 132

Mexican Chicken Salad 135

Nori Wrapped Fish 138

Roasted Acorn Squash 141

Vegetable Fruit Plate 144

Herbed Fish Veggies 146

Roasted Fish with Veggies 149

Salmon Veggies 152

Grilled Burger 154

Veggie Strips with Guacamole 157

Conclusion 159

About the Author.. 160

Author's Afterthoughts.. 161

Introduction

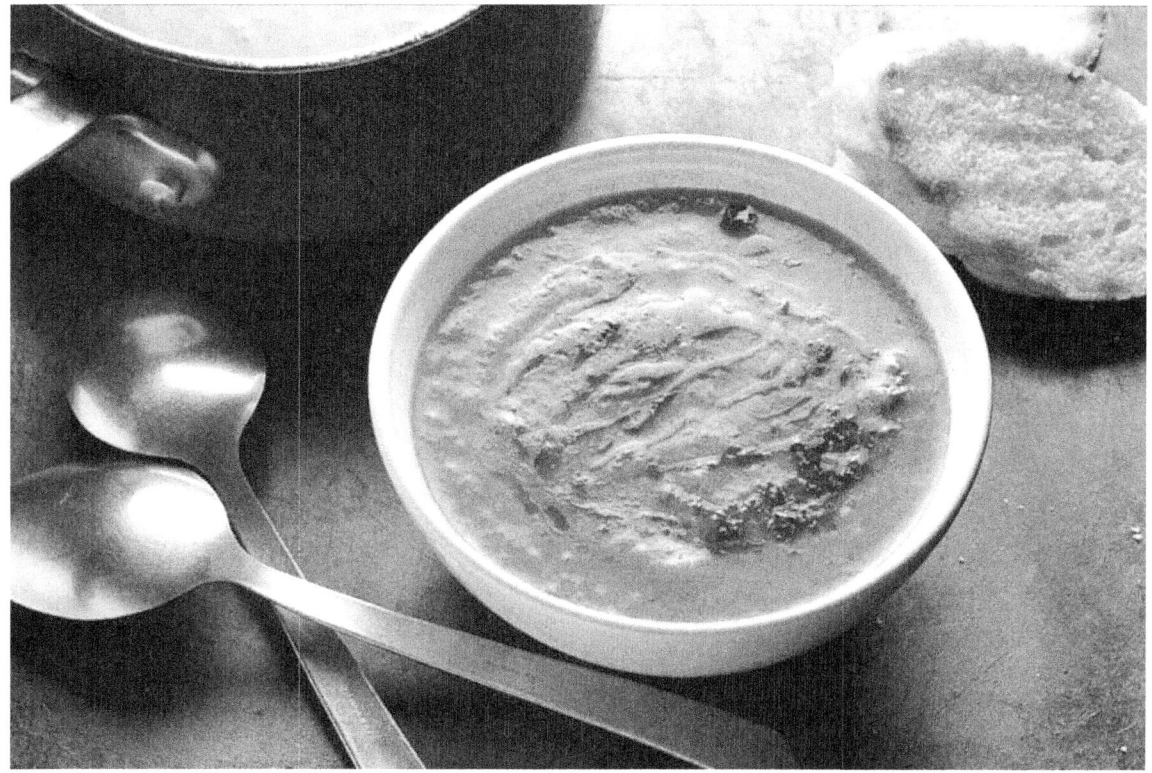

According to the World Health Organization (WHO), more than 1 billion people worldwide suffer from high blood pressure. And in the United States, up to 103 million have hypertension, as reported by the American Heart Association.

High blood pressure can actually exist without any symptoms; some people are not aware until they already suffered from life-threatening complications. So, because of this condition, hypertension has been called a "silent killer."

Aside from getting regular checkups to monitor one's blood pressure levels, it is of utmost importance to lead a healthy lifestyle, a significant facet of which is a proper diet.

For people who already were diagnosed as hypertension, most doctors recommend the "DASH" diet.

DASH is short for Dietary Approaches to Stop Hypertension.

Basically, one must follow these guidelines to manage blood pressure levels:

- Consume more fruits and vegetables.
- Eat more fish and seafood.
- Minimize the consumption of foods high in fats and cholesterol.
- Tone down intake of sodium and sugar.
- Limit intake of red meat and processed food products.
- Include more whole grains and healthy fats.

The research has shown that people who take on the DASH diet, the blood pressure levels improve in 2 weeks.

In this book, you will find recipes that are not only low in fat and cholesterol, but also sugar and sodium.

These recipes are not only advisable when you're already suffering from hypertension, but these recipes can also help you to prevent the condition.

Take a step towards healthier living today.

Scallop Salad

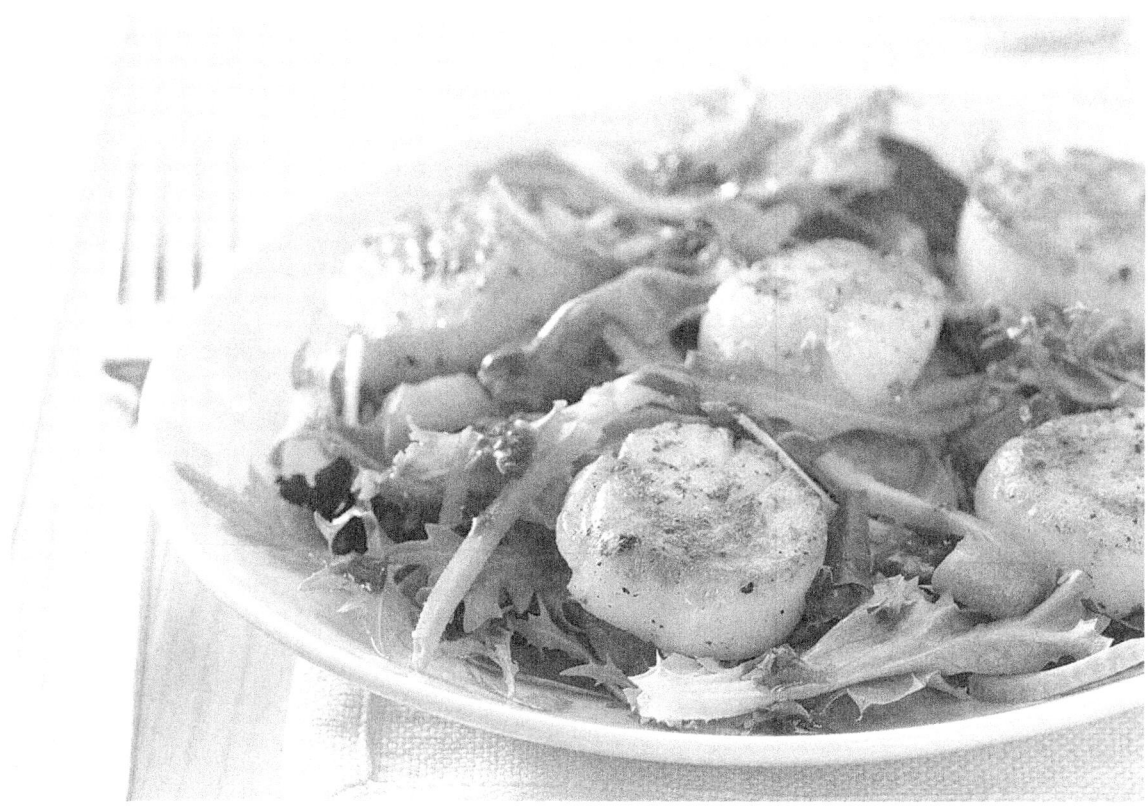

Leafy greens topped with seared scallops and served with chopped tomatoes, cucumber, and corn create a light but delicious meal that's perfect for brunch or lunch.

Serving Size: 4

Preparation Cooking Time: 30 minutes

Ingredients:

- ¼ cup fresh basil leaves, chopped
- 2 tablespoons freshly squeezed lemon juice
- 3 tablespoons balsamic vinegar
- 2 teaspoons Dijon mustard
- 2 tablespoons olive oil
- Pepper to taste
- 1 lb. scallops
- 6 cups salad greens, chopped
- 1 English cucumber, chopped
- 1 cup corn kernels
- 1 red bell pepper, chopped
- 3 tomatoes, seeded and chopped
- 2 tablespoons Parmesan cheese, grated

Instructions:

1. Mix the basil, lemon juice, vinegar, mustard, olive oil and pepper in a glass jar with lid.

2. Shake the jar. Put it in the refrigerator.

3. Season the scallops with the pepper.

4. Spray your pan with oil.

5. Put it over medium high heat.

6. Cook the scallops for 2 minutes per side.

7. Arrange the salad greens on serving plates.

8. In a bowl, combine the cucumber, corn kernels, red bell pepper and tomatoes.

9. Pour in half of the basil mixture to the cucumber mixture.

10. Toss to coat evenly.

11. Add the scallops on top of the leafy greens.

12. Pour with the remaining basil mixture.

13. Serve with the corn salsa and sprinkle with the Parmesan cheese.

Nutrients per Serving:

- Calories 261
- Fat 9.2 g
- Saturated fat 1.6 g
- Carbohydrates 21.4 g
- Fiber 3.8 g
- Protein 23.4 g
- Cholesterol 39 mg
- Sugars 8 g
- Sodium 282 mg
- Potassium 845 mg

Salmon Satay

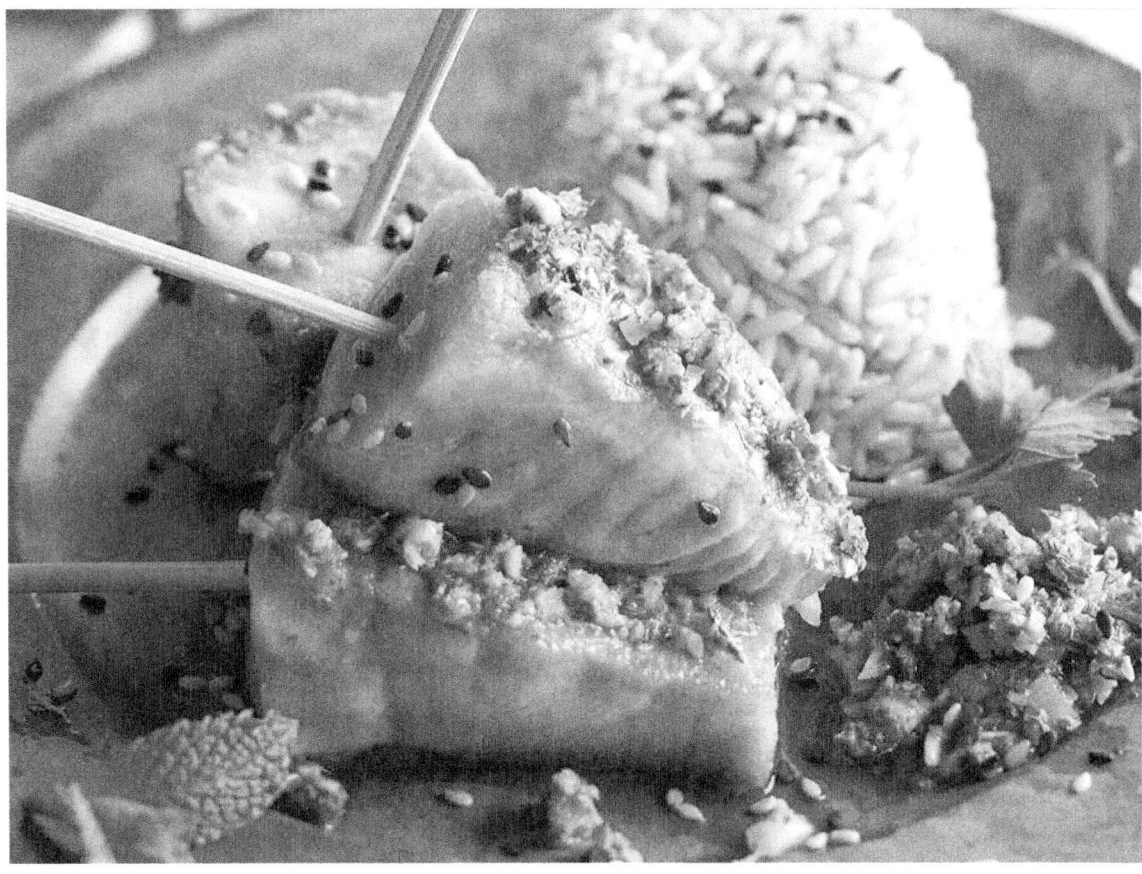

Sear your salmon cubes and spread with Asian style pesto (made of mint, ginger, lemongrass, and parsley). This goes perfectly with brown rice or salad.

Serving Size: 4

Preparation Cooking Time: 45 minutes

Ingredients:

- 5 teaspoons vegetable oil, divided
- 1 tablespoon onion, chopped
- 1 cup uncooked brown rice
- 1 ½ cups low-sodium chicken stock
- 16 oz. salmon fillet, sliced into large cubes
- 2 teaspoons black sesame seeds, toasted
- 4 sprigs fresh mint, chopped
- 4 sprigs fresh cilantro, chopped
- 4 sprigs fresh Italian parsley

Pesto

- 1 tablespoon vegetable oil
- ½ teaspoon toasted sesame oil
- 3 cloves garlic, peeled
- 2 tablespoons freshly squeezed lime juice
- ¼ cup fresh Italian parsley leaves
- ¾ cup fresh mint leaves
- 2 tablespoons fresh lemongrass
- 2 teaspoons freshly grated ginger
- 1 chili pepper, chopped
- Salt to taste

Instructions:

1. Pour 2 teaspoons vegetable oil into a pan over medium heat.

2. Cook the onion for 3 minutes.

3. Stir in the brown rice and stock.

4. Bring to a boil.

5. Reduce heat and simmer for 45 minutes.

6. Set aside.

7. Brush the salmon cubes with the remaining oil.

8. Thread onto skewers.

9. Grill for 2 to 3 minutes per side.

10. Add all the pesto ingredients in the food processor.

11. Pulse until smooth.

12. Spread the pesto on top of the salmon.

13. Serve with the brown rice.

14. Sprinkle with the sesame seeds.

15. Garnish with the herb sprigs.

Nutrients per Serving:

- Calories 401
- Fat 18.5 g
- Saturated fat 2.4 g
- Carbohydrates 30.4 g
- Fiber 2.2 g
- Protein 27.3 g
- Cholesterol 62 mg
- Sugars 1 g
- Sodium 412 mg
- Potassium 809 mg

Salmon Tostadas

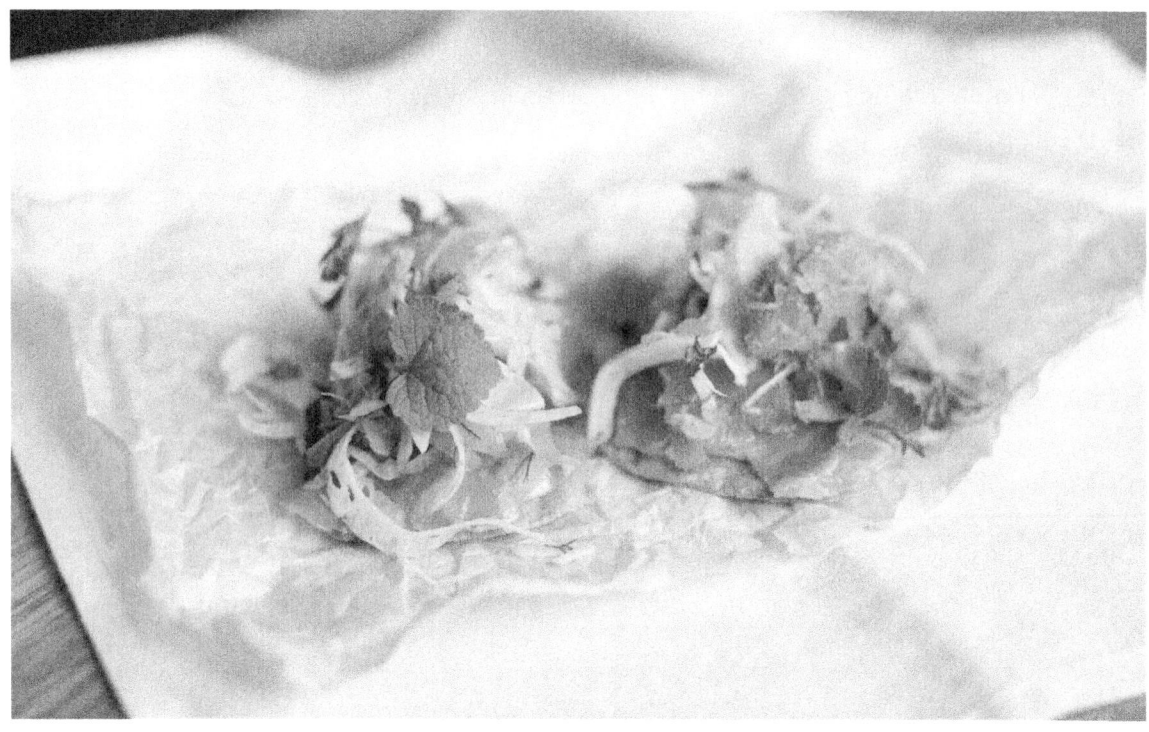

Create a nutritious and satisfying meal with this citrus-marinated salmon served with kale and creamy avocado chunks and rolled into tortillas.

Serving Size: 4

Preparation Cooking Time: 1 hour and 40 minutes

Ingredients:

- ¼ cup lime juice
- ½ cup orange juice
- ½ teaspoon chili powder
- Pepper to taste
- 1 lb. salmon fillets
- 1 ripe avocado, sliced into chunks and divided
- ½ cup scallions, chopped
- 1 teaspoon olive oil
- 2 teaspoons honey
- Salt to taste
- 4 cups kale, chopped
- 4 tortillas, toasted

Instructions:

1. Make the marinade by mixing the lime juice, orange juice, chili powder and pepper in a bowl.

2. Soak the salmon and cover with foil.

3. Chill in the refrigerator for 30 minutes.

4. Preheat your oven to 400 degrees F.

5. Add half of the avocado, scallions, oil, honey and salt in your food processor.

6. Pulse until smooth.

7. Toss the kale and avocado in the avocado dressing.

8. Add the salmon with marinade in a pan over medium heat.

9. Simmer for 12 minutes.

10. Top the tortillas with the salmon and kale mixture.

11. Roll up the tortillas.

Nutrients per Serving:

- Calories 419
- Fat 16.6 g
- Saturated fat 3.8 g
- Carbohydrates 37.3 g
- Fiber 17.3 g
- Protein 33.3 g
- Cholesterol 60 mg
- Sugars 8 g
- Sodium 505 mg
- Potassium 1033 mg

Sirloin Salad

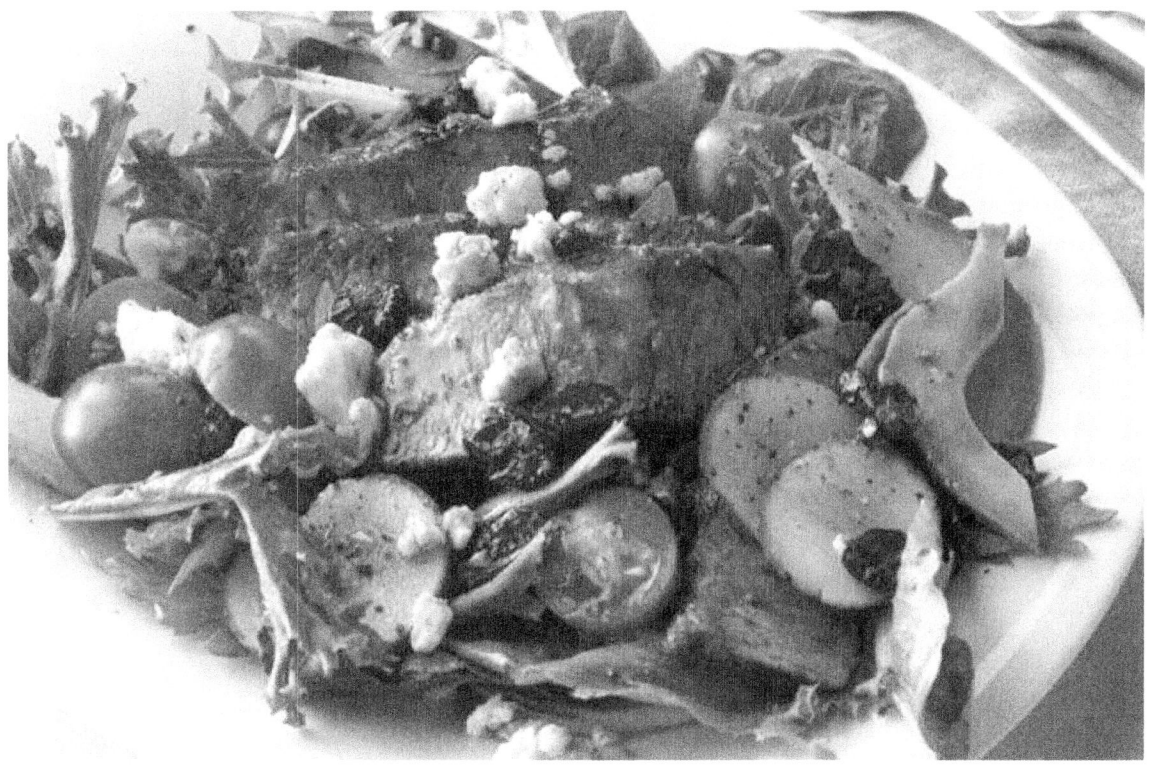

Just because you're monitoring your blood pressure levels, it doesn't mean that you cannot enjoy beef again. With this recipe, you can make yourself a light and delicious dish—beef salad with arugula, onions, corn kernels and, beef sirloin strips.

Serving Size: 4

Preparation Cooking Time: 1 hour

Ingredients:

- ¼ teaspoon ground cinnamon
- 1 tablespoon instant coffee granules
- Salt and pepper to taste
- 1 lb. beef sirloin steak, fat trimmed
- 1 cup corn kernels
- 2 teaspoons canola oil
- ¼ cup balsamic vinegar
- 1 ½ teaspoons sugar
- ¼ cup dry red wine
- 4 cups arugula
- 1 chili pepper, sliced thinly
- 16 cherry tomatoes, sliced in half
- ¼ cup red onion, sliced thinly

Instructions:

1. Combine the cinnamon, coffee, salt and pepper in a bowl.

2. Coat both sides of the beef with this mixture.

3. Marinate for 15 minutes.

4. Add the corn kernels in a pan over medium heat.

5. Cook for 3 minutes.

6. Transfer to a plate.

7. Pour the oil in the same pan and add the beef.

8. Cook for 10 minutes, flipping once or twice.

9. Transfer to a plate.

10. Add the vinegar, sugar and vinegar to the same pan.

11. Bring to a boil.

12. Simmer until sauce is reduced.

13. Remove from the stove.

14. Top the arugula with the beef and sprinkle the tomatoes, onions and chili pepper on top.

Nutrients per Serving:

- Calories 283
- Fat 7.6 g
- Saturated fat 2 g
- Carbohydrates 21.5 g
- Fiber 2.4 g
- Protein 28.3 g
- Cholesterol 48 mg
- Sugars 8 g
- Sodium 154 mg
- Potassium 900 mg

Zucchini Noodles with Pesto

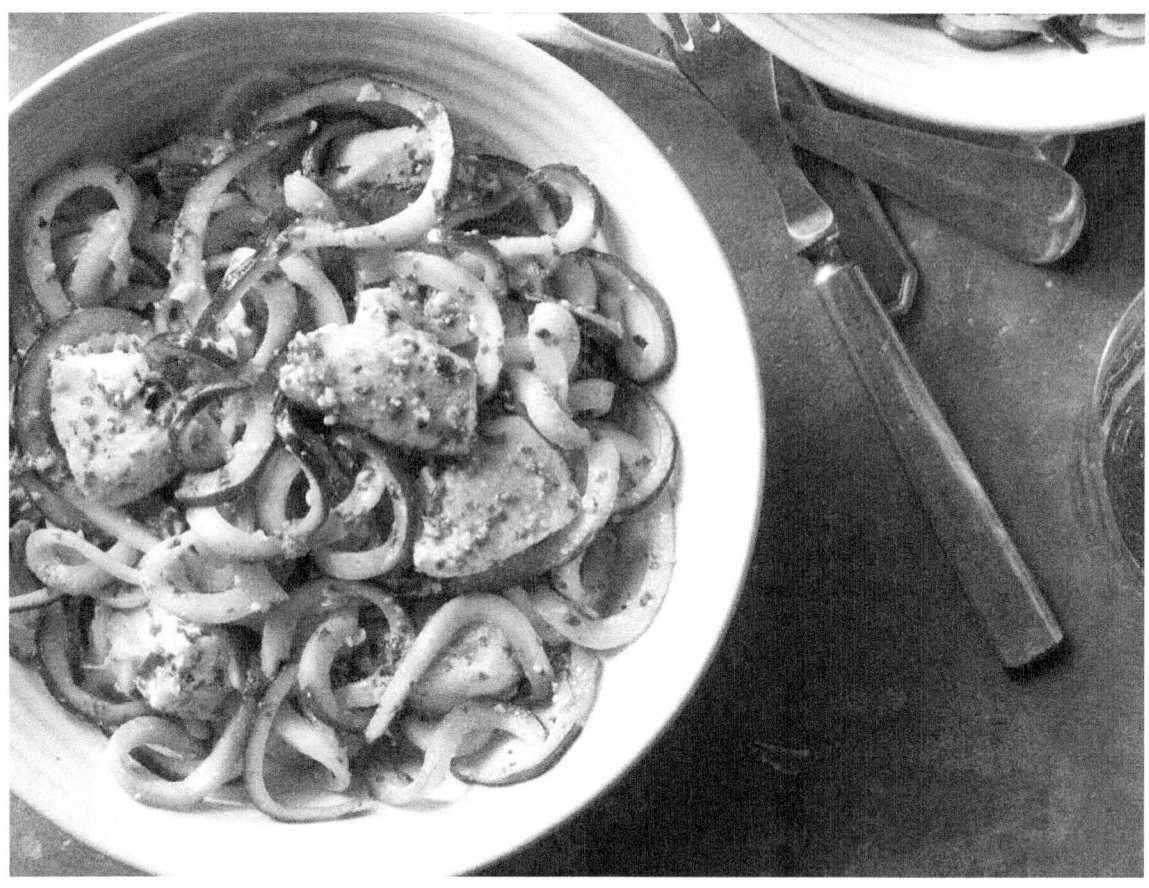

This pesto pasta makes by using the zucchini noodles, topped with almonds and tomatoes.

Serving Size: 6

Preparation Cooking Time: 40 minutes

Ingredients:

- 2 zucchini, spiralized
- Salt to taste
- ½ cup almonds, toasted
- 3 cups cherry tomatoes
- 3 cloves garlic
- 1 cup fresh basil
- ¼ teaspoon red pepper flakes
- 3 tablespoons olive oil, divided
- 8 oz. whole-wheat spaghetti
- 1 lb. salmon fillets
- Pepper to taste

Instructions:

1. Boil the zucchini noodles in a pot with water.

2. Drain in a colander.

3. Season with the salt.

4. Let sit for 20 minutes.

5. Add the almonds in a food processor.

6. Pulse until chopped.

7. Add the tomatoes, garlic, basil leaves and red pepper flakes.

8. Pulse until well combined.

9. Pour in 2 tablespoons oil and salt.

10. Pulse until smooth.

11. Prepare the spaghetti according to the directions in the package. Drain.

12. Add the remaining oil in a pan over medium heat.

13. Sprinkle the salmon with the salt and pepper.

14. Cook the salmon in the pan for 3 minutes per side.

15. Use a fork to flake the salmon.

16. Toss the spaghetti in the salmon and pesto.

17. Sprinkle with the Parmesan cheese and serve.

Nutrients per Serving:

- Calories 450
- Fat 23.5 g
- Saturated fat 3.8 g
- Carbohydrates 40.8 g
- Fiber 7.1 g
- Protein 25.9 g
- Cholesterol 42 mg
- Sugars 5 g
- Sodium 459 mg
- Potassium 816 mg

Pistachio Crusted Mahi Mahi

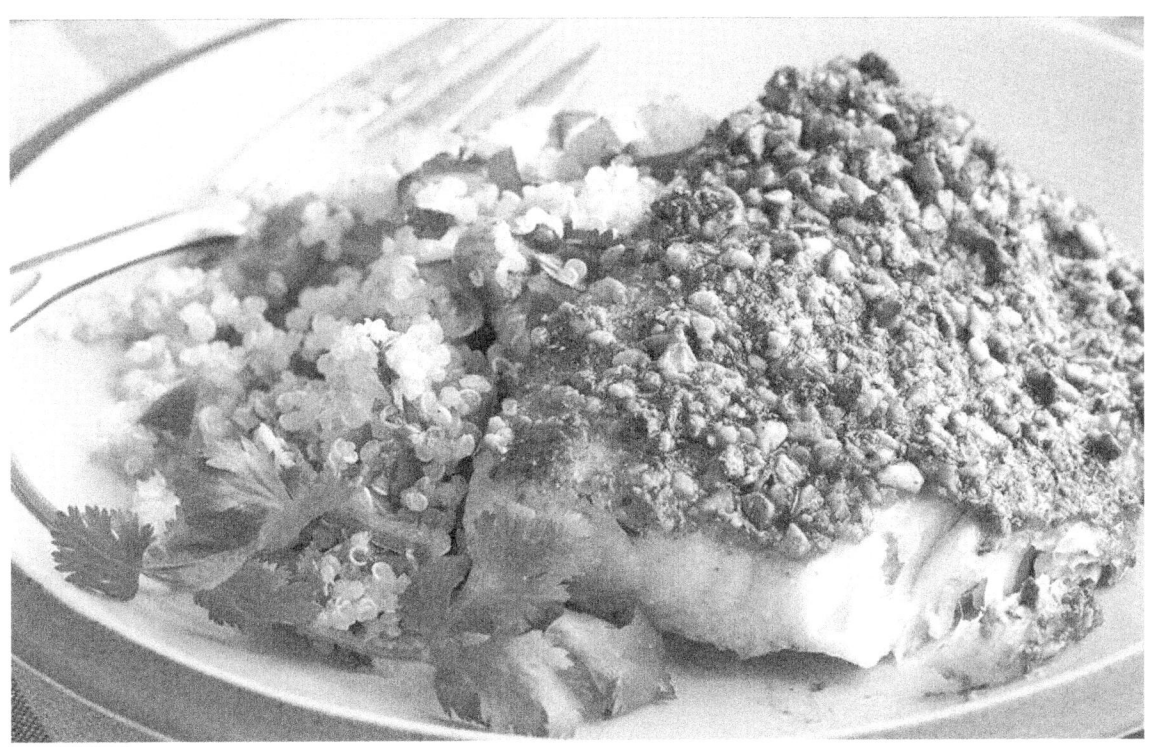

Coat your mahi mahi with pistachio and chili breading to create a fusion of nutty and spicy flavors. For sure, this will become a hit at the dinner table.

Serving Size: 4

Preparation Cooking Time: 45 minutes

Ingredients:

- 1 tablespoon lime juice
- 1 teaspoon lime zest
- Salt and pepper to taste
- 2 teaspoons olive oil
- 5 teaspoons honey, divided
- ½ cup pistachio, roasted
- ¼ teaspoon paprika
- ¼ teaspoon onion powder
- ¾ teaspoon chili powder
- 4 mahi mahi fillets
- 1 ¼ cups cooked quinoa
- ¼ cup onion, chopped
- ¼ cup fresh cilantro leaves, chopped
- ½ cup red bell pepper, chopped

Instructions:

1. Preheat your oven to 325 degrees F.

2. Line your baking pan with parchment paper.

3. Combine the lime juice, lime zest, salt, pepper, olive oil and 2 teaspoons honey in a bowl. Set aside.

4. In another bowl, mix 1 teaspoon honey, pistachios, paprika, onion powder and chili powder.

5. Spread this mixture on a baking pan.

6. Bake in the oven for 12 minutes.

7. Transfer the mixture to a food processor.

8. Pulse until crushed.

9. Increase temperature of oven to 425 degrees F.

10. Brush the fish with the remaining honey.

11. Coat both sides with the pistachio mixture.

12. Press to adhere.

13. Put the fish on the baking pan.

14. Bake for 15 minutes.

15. In a bowl, combine the rest of the ingredients.

16. Add the lime dressing to the quinoa mixture.

17. Serve the mahi mahi with the quinoa mixture.

Nutrients per Serving:

- Calories 322
- Fat 11.5 g
- Saturated fat 1.6 g
- Carbohydrates 28.3 g
- Fiber 4.3 g
- Protein 27.5 g
- Cholesterol 83 mg
- Sugars 10 g
- Sodium 328 mg
- Potassium 829 mg

Creamy Tomato Soup

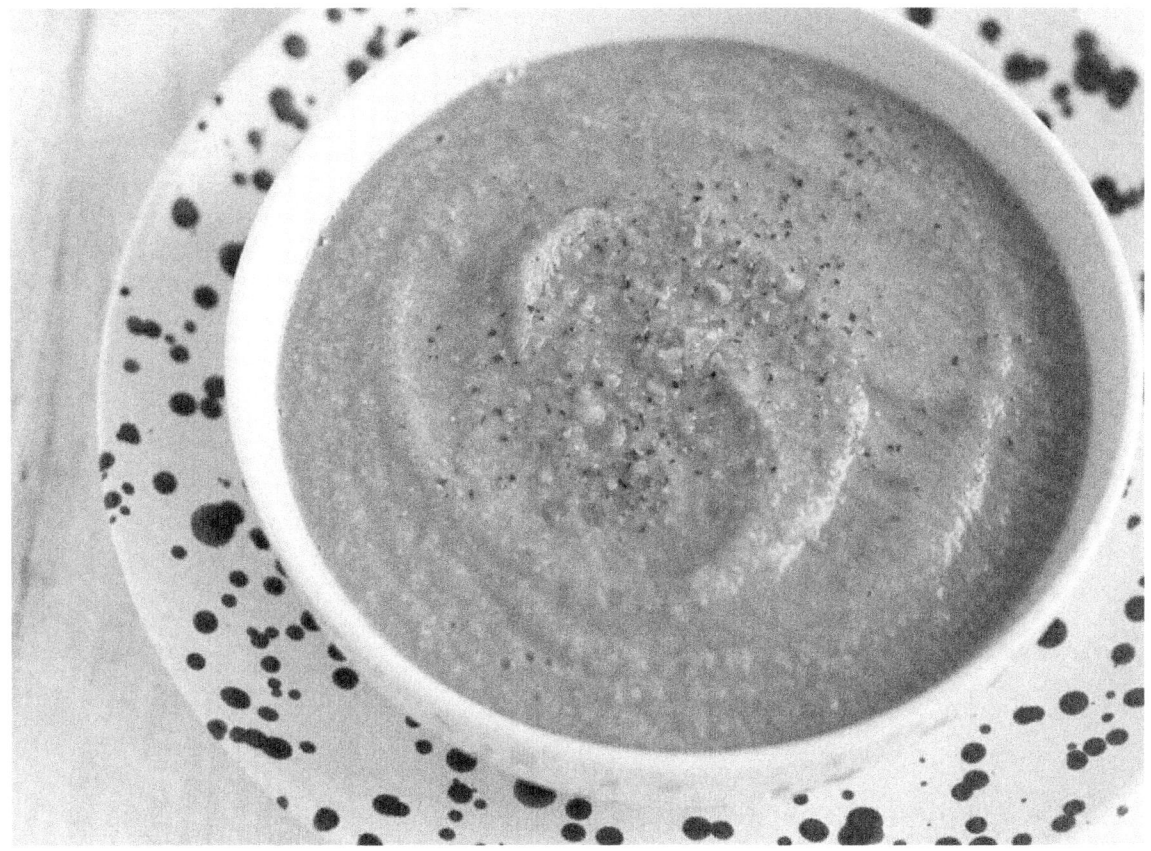

Simmer up this creamy tomato soup to brighten up a gloomy day. This nourishing soup, which is made only with three ingredients—tomato puree, cream cheese, and chicken broth—brings comfort with every sip.

Serving Size: 1

Preparation Cooking Time: 5 minutes

Ingredients:

- 1 cup tomato puree (unsalted)
- ¼ cup reduced-sodium chicken broth
- 1 tablespoon low-fat cream cheese

Instructions:

1. Combine the three ingredients in a microwave-friendly mug.

2. Microwave on high for 2 minutes.

3. Stir and serve.

Nutrients per Serving:

- Calories 105
- Fat 2.7 g
- Saturated fat 1.4 g
- Carbohydrates 18.3 g
- Fiber 3.6 g
- Protein 5.1 g
- Cholesterol 8 mg
- Sugars 10 g
- Sodium 245 mg
- Potassium 911 mg

Pesto Penne with Chicken Veggies

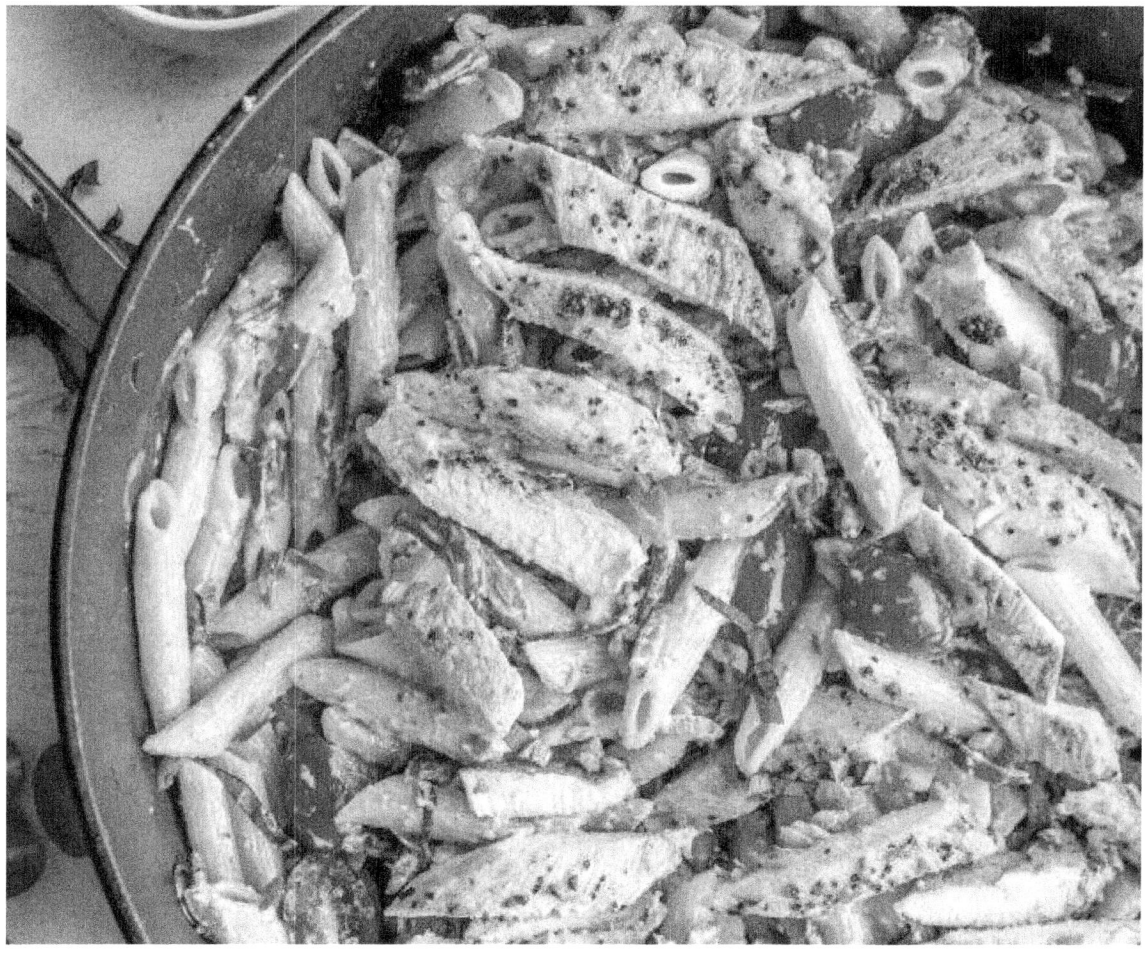

For tonight's dinner, eliminate all the hard work by opting for this incredibly easy pasta recipe that's made with chicken and vegetables. It has all the flavors you love, but there's no need to worry about your blood pressure levels.

Serving Size: 4

Preparation Cooking Time: 30 minutes

Ingredients:

- ¾ cup walnuts, chopped
- Salt and pepper to taste
- 2 cloves garlic, peeled and crushed
- 1 cup parsley leaves
- 2 tablespoons olive oil
- ¼ cup Parmesan cheese, grated
- 8 oz. chicken breast, cooked and shredded
- 6 oz. whole-wheat penne
- 8 oz. green beans, sliced and steamed
- 2 cups cauliflower florets, steamed

Instructions:

1. Add half of the walnuts to a bowl.

2. Toast the walnuts in a pan over medium heat for 2 minutes.

3. Place these on a plate and let cool.

4. Add the remaining walnuts in the food processor along with the salt, pepper, garlic and parsley.

5. Pulse until fully ground.

6. Gradually pour in the oil.

7. Stir in the Parmesan cheese.

8. Pulse until fully combined.

9. Add the pesto to a bowl.

10. Stir in the chicken.

11. Prepare the pasta according to package directions.

12. Drain the pasta.

13. Add the pasta to the pesto and chicken mixture.

14. Top with the toasted walnuts and serve.

Nutrients per Serving:

- Calories 514
- Fat 26.6 g
- Saturated fat 4.2 g
- Carbohydrates 43.4 g
- Fiber 8.6 g
- Protein 31.4 g
- Cholesterol 54 mg
- Sugars 5 g
- Sodium 557 mg
- Potassium 817 mg

Lettuce Wraps

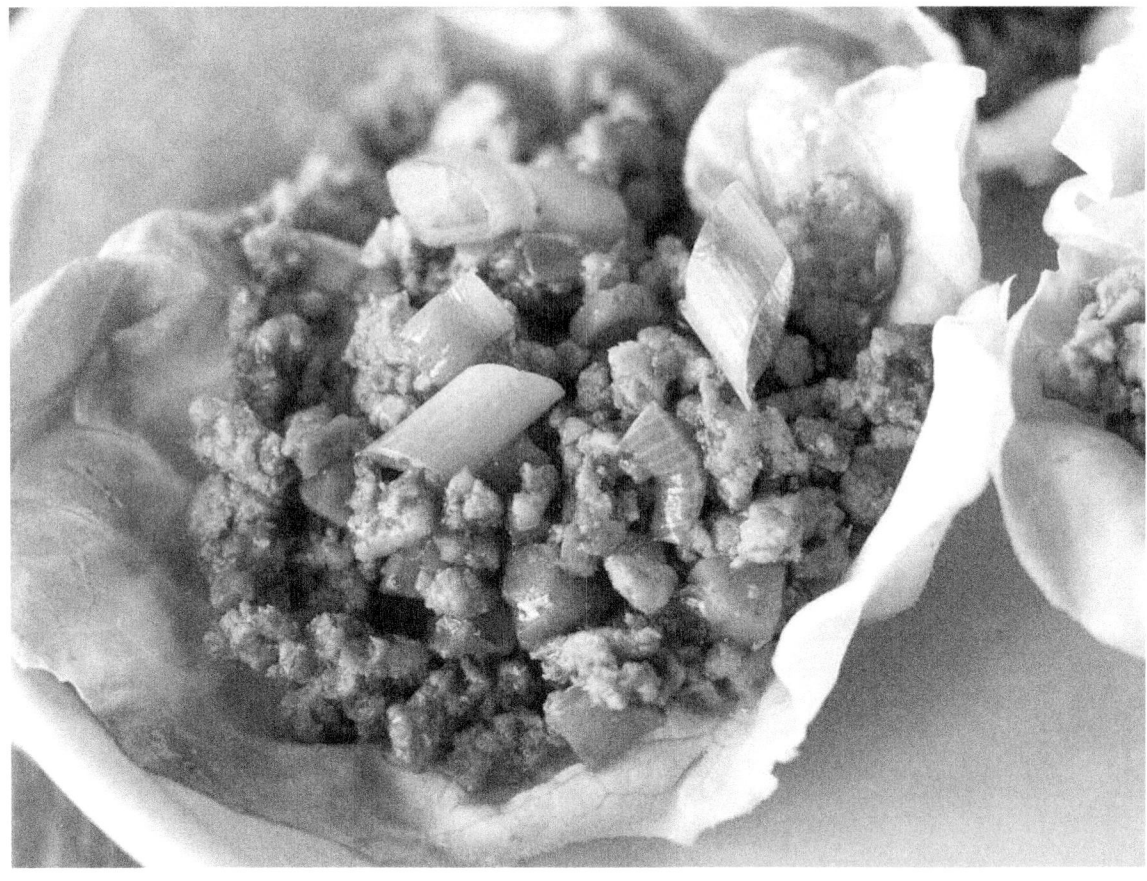

This is just one of the many exciting ways to prepare lettuce—top it with a salad made of beans, chickpeas, and quinoa!

Serving Size: 4

Preparation Cooking Time: 10 minutes

Ingredients:

Salad

- 1 clove garlic, minced
- Salt to taste
- 30 oz. kidney beans, rinsed and drained
- 15 oz. chickpeas, rinsed and drained
- ½ cup olive oil
- ¼ cup freshly squeezed lemon juice
- 2 tablespoons ground cumin
- ¼ teaspoon ground cinnamon
- 1 cup carrot, chopped
- 1 ½ cups parsley, chopped
- ½ cup fresh mint leaves, chopped

Lettuce Wraps

- 2 heads lettuce
- 1 ½ cups cooked quinoa
- ¼ cup fresh mint leaves

Instructions:

1. Mash the garlic with a fork or knife.

2. Sprinkle with the salt and mix to form a paste.

3. Add the pasta to a bowl.

4. Add the rest of the salad ingredients. Mix well.

5. Top each lettuce leaf with the salad, quinoa and mint leaves.

6. Roll and serve.

Nutrients per Serving:

- Calories 425
- Fat 19.8 g
- Saturated fat 2.7 g
- Carbohydrates 50.1 g
- Fiber 14.4 g
- Protein 13.7 g
- Cholesterol 10 mg
- Sugars 3 g
- Sodium 551 mg
- Potassium 871 mg

Shrimp with Artichoke Salad

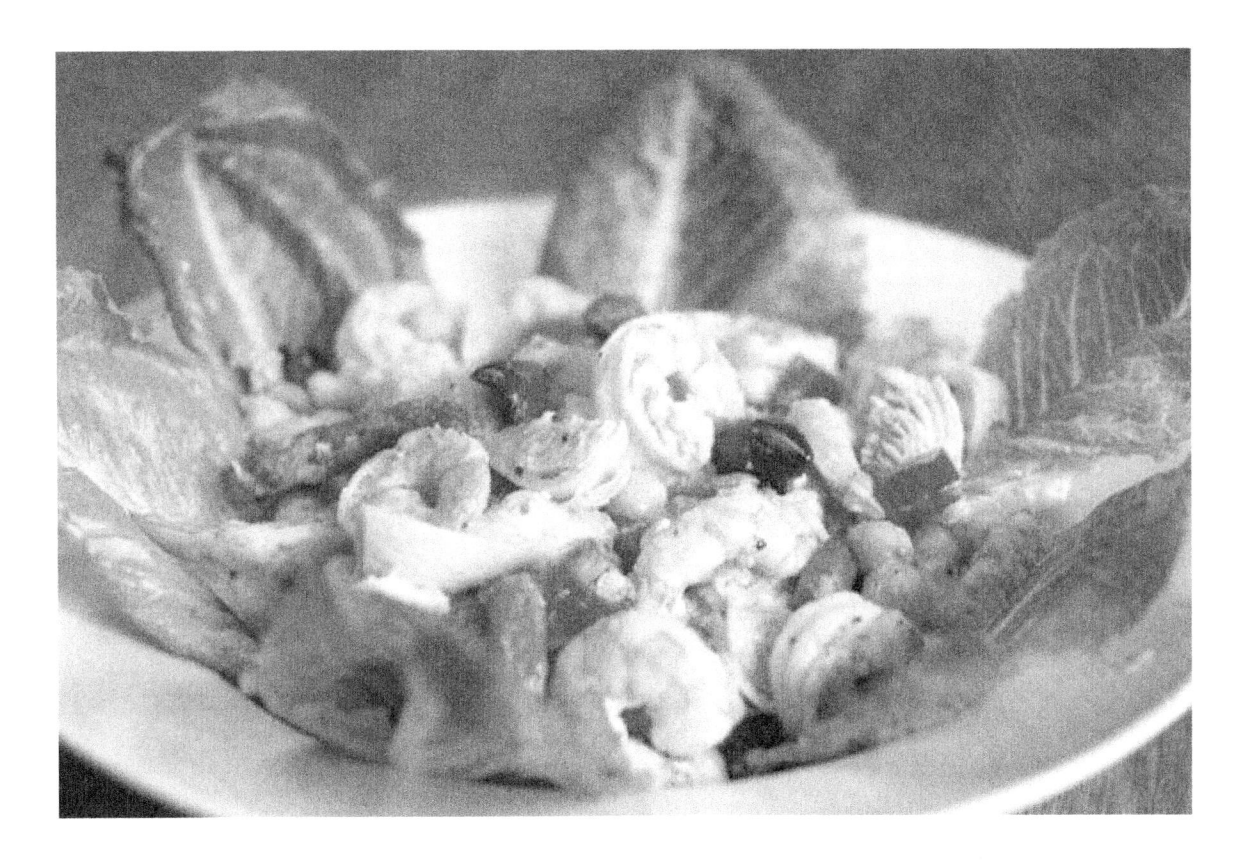

This healthy salad is perfect for family dinners, backyard parties, small gatherings, and so on. This only takes a few minutes to prepare.

Serving Size: 4

Preparation Cooking Time: 1 hour

Ingredients:

- 1 tablespoon lemon juice
- 1 tablespoon water
- 12 artichokes, trimmed and sliced
- 4 tablespoons olive oil, divided
- Salt and pepper to taste
- 2 tablespoons fresh mint leaves
- ½ lb. shrimp, deveined

Instructions:

1. Soak the artichokes in lemon juice and water.

2. Drain.

3. Mix half of the oil, salt, pepper and mint leaves in a bowl.

4. Toss the artichokes in this mixture.

5. Pour the remaining oil in a pan over medium heat.

6. Cook the shrimp for 3 minutes, sprinkling with salt and pepper.

7. Serve with the artichokes.

Nutrients per Serving:

- Calories 243
- Fat 14.4 g
- Saturated fat 2 g
- Carbohydrates 18.3 g
- Fiber 9.4 g
- Protein 14.3 g
- Cholesterol 68 mg
- Sugars 2 g
- Sodium 237 mg
- Potassium 737 mg

Turkey Burger

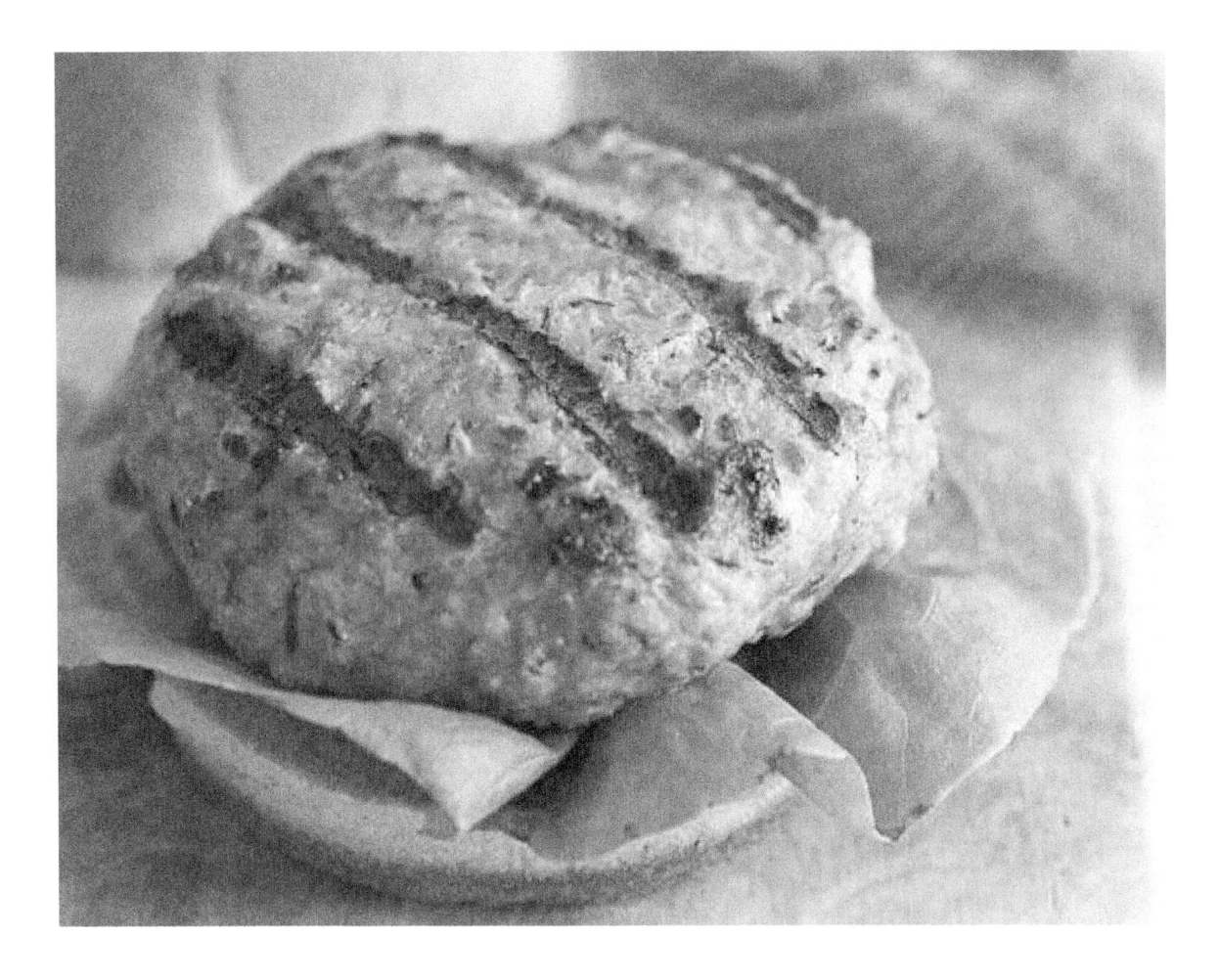

Craving for burger but worried about what fats can do to your health? Create the patty by using lean ground turkey instead of beef and make of Portobello mushrooms as buns. The result is truly unforgettable.

Serving Size: 4

Preparation Cooking Time: 30 minutes

Ingredients:

- 2 tablespoons olive oil
- Salt and pepper to taste
- 1 clove garlic, crushed and minced
- 8 Portobello mushroom caps, gill and stems removed
- 1 lb. lean ground turkey
- 1 teaspoon Dijon mustard
- 2 teaspoons Worcestershire sauce
- 4 slices Swiss cheese
- 3 cups arugula
- 1 tomato, sliced thinly

Instructions:

1. Preheat your grill.

2. In a bowl, combine the oil, salt, pepper and garlic.

3. Brush the mushroom caps with this mixture.

4. Marinate for 10 minutes.

5. In another bowl, mix the ground turkey, salt, pepper, mustard and Worcestershire sauce.

6. Form 4 patties from the mixture.

7. Grill the mushrooms for 4 minutes per side.

8. Transfer to a plate.

9. Add the turkey patties and grill for 5 minutes per side.

10. Place the cheese slices on top of the turkey patties and grill for 1 more minute.

11. Top each of the mushroom caps with the arugula and tomato slices.

12. Add the turkey patty with cheese.

13. Cover with the remaining mushroom caps.

Nutrients per Serving:

- Calories 332
- Fat 18.4 g
- Saturated fat 4.4 g
- Carbohydrates 10.3 g
- Fiber 2.9 g
- Protein 33.5 g
- Cholesterol 94 mg
- Sugars 6 g
- Sodium 503 mg
- Potassium 1046 mg

Baked Chicken Asparagus

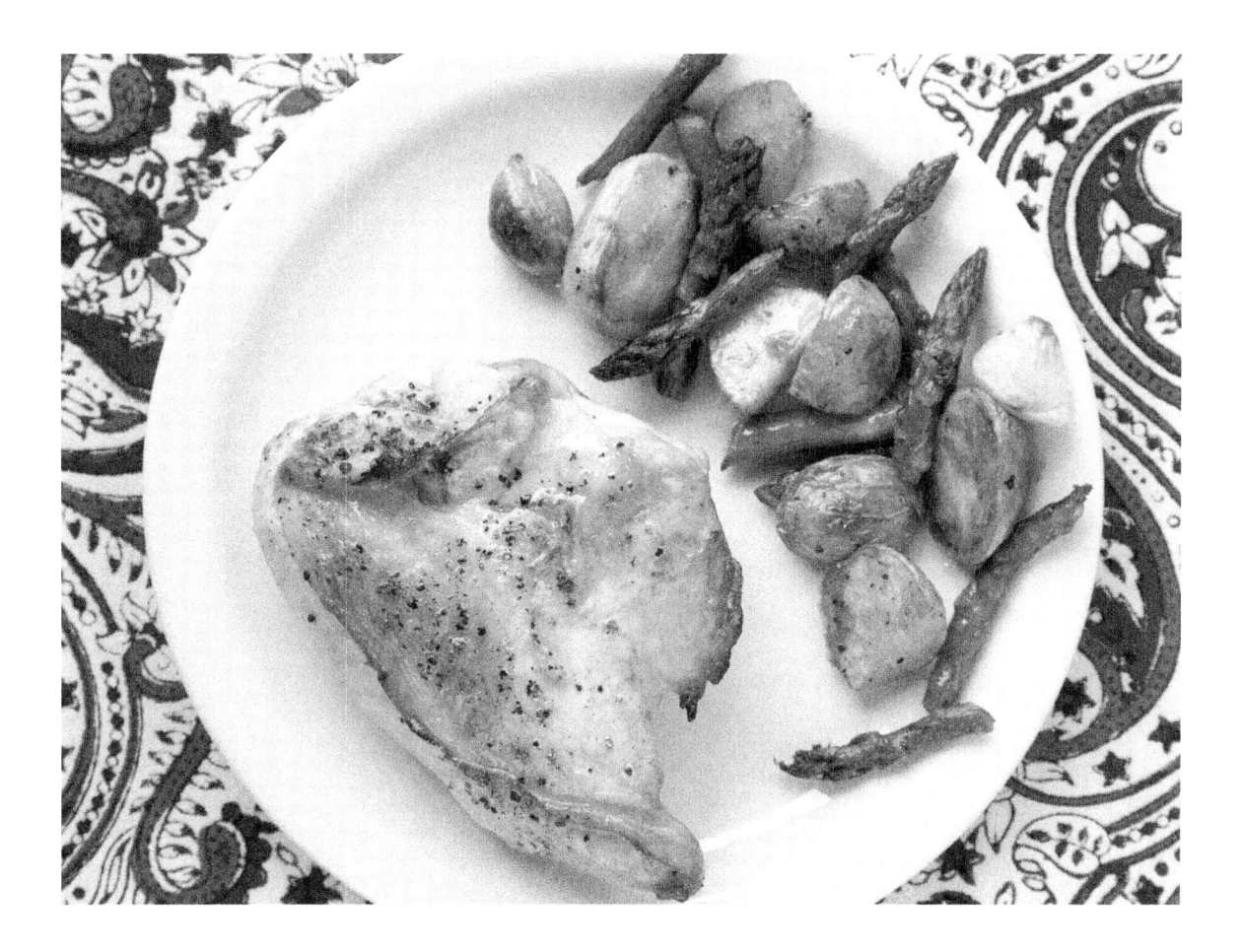

When you're managing hypertension with proper diet, baked dishes are some of your best choices. These usually have lesser fat and calories than deep-fried. But it doesn't mean you have to sacrifice flavor. Here's a baked chicken and asparagus recipe that you won't regret preparing for yourself and your family.

Serving Size: 4

Preparation Cooking Time: 35 minutes

Ingredients:

- 16 chicken breast fillet
- 8 oz. carrots, sliced
- 12 oz. baby potatoes, sliced in half
- 3 tablespoons olive oil, divided
- 2 teaspoons ground coriander, divided
- Salt and pepper to taste
- 2 tablespoons shallot, chopped
- 2 teaspoons honey
- 2 tablespoons lemon juice
- 1 tablespoon mustard
- 1 lb. fresh asparagus, trimmed
- 1 tablespoon fresh dill, chopped
- 2 tablespoons parsley, chopped

Instructions:

1. Preheat your oven to 375 degrees F.

2. Wrap the chicken with cling wrap.

3. Pound the chicken with a meat mallet to flatten.

4. Place the chicken on one side of a baking pan.

5. In a bowl, toss the carrots and potatoes, and place on the other side of the pan.

6. Drizzle the veggies and chicken with 1 tablespoon oil and sprinkle with half of the paprika.

7. Season with the salt and pepper.

8. Bake in the oven for 15 minutes.

9. In another bowl, combine the remaining oil, remaining coriander, salt, pepper, shallot, honey, lemon juice and mustard.

10. Stir into the pan the asparagus.

11. Drizzle the mustard mixture on top of the chicken and veggies.

12. Bake for 10 minutes.

13. Sprinkle the dill and parsley on top.

Nutrients per Serving:

- Calories 352
- Fat 13.8 g
- Saturated fat 2.3 g
- Carbohydrates 30.7 g
- Fiber 5.7 g
- Protein 27.6 g
- Cholesterol 63 mg
- Sugars 8 g
- Sodium 599 mg
- Potassium 910 mg

Baked Tuna Steak

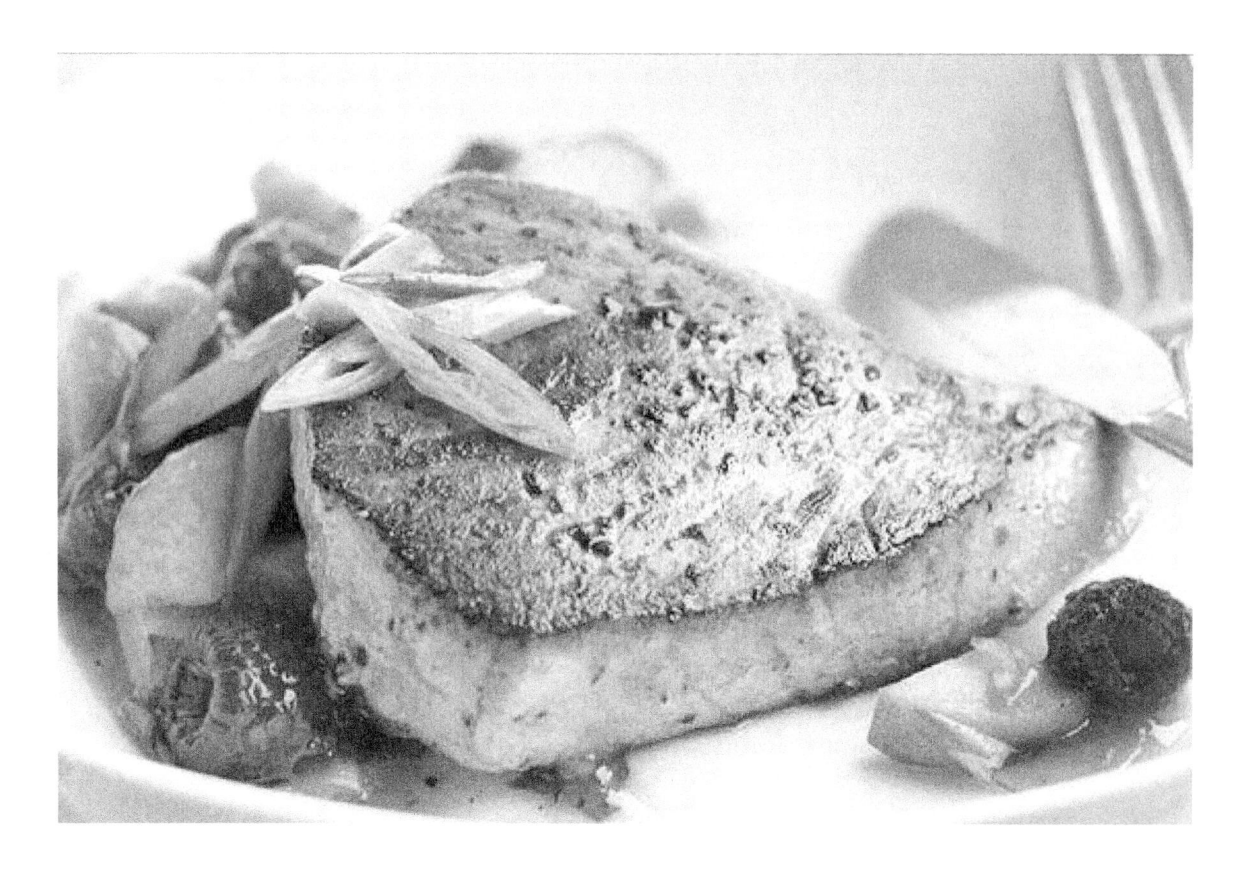

Here's another baked recipe that's low in fat and calories but doesn't disappoint when it comes to flavor.

Serving Size: 4

Preparation Cooking Time: 30 minutes

Ingredients:

- ¼ cup mayonnaise
- 1 teaspoon honey
- 2 teaspoons Dijon mustard
- ½ teaspoon ground turmeric
- 1 tablespoon parsley, chopped
- 2 cups potatoes, sliced thinly
- Salt and pepper to taste
- 4 cups kale, chopped
- 1 ¼ lb. tuna steaks

Instructions:

1. Preheat your oven to 450 degrees F.

2. Line your baking pan with parchment paper.

3. In a bowl, mix the mayonnaise, honey, mustard, turmeric and parsley.

4. Season the potatoes with the salt and pepper.

5. Lay 4 sheets of foil on your kitchen table.

6. Place 1 slice tuna and 1 cup kale on top of each foil.

7. Season with the salt and pepper.

8. Spread the mayo mixture on top.

9. Cover the tuna and place the foil packets on the baking pan.

10. Bake for 12 to 15 minutes.

11. Let sit for 3 minutes before serving.

Nutrients per Serving:

- Calories 312
- Fat 11.3 g
- Saturated fat 1.9 g
- Carbohydrates 14 g
- Fiber 1.7 g
- Protein 36.4 g
- Cholesterol 61 mg
- Sugars 2 g
- Sodium 512 mg
- Potassium 901 mg

Sweet Potatoes Stuffed with Chicken Curry

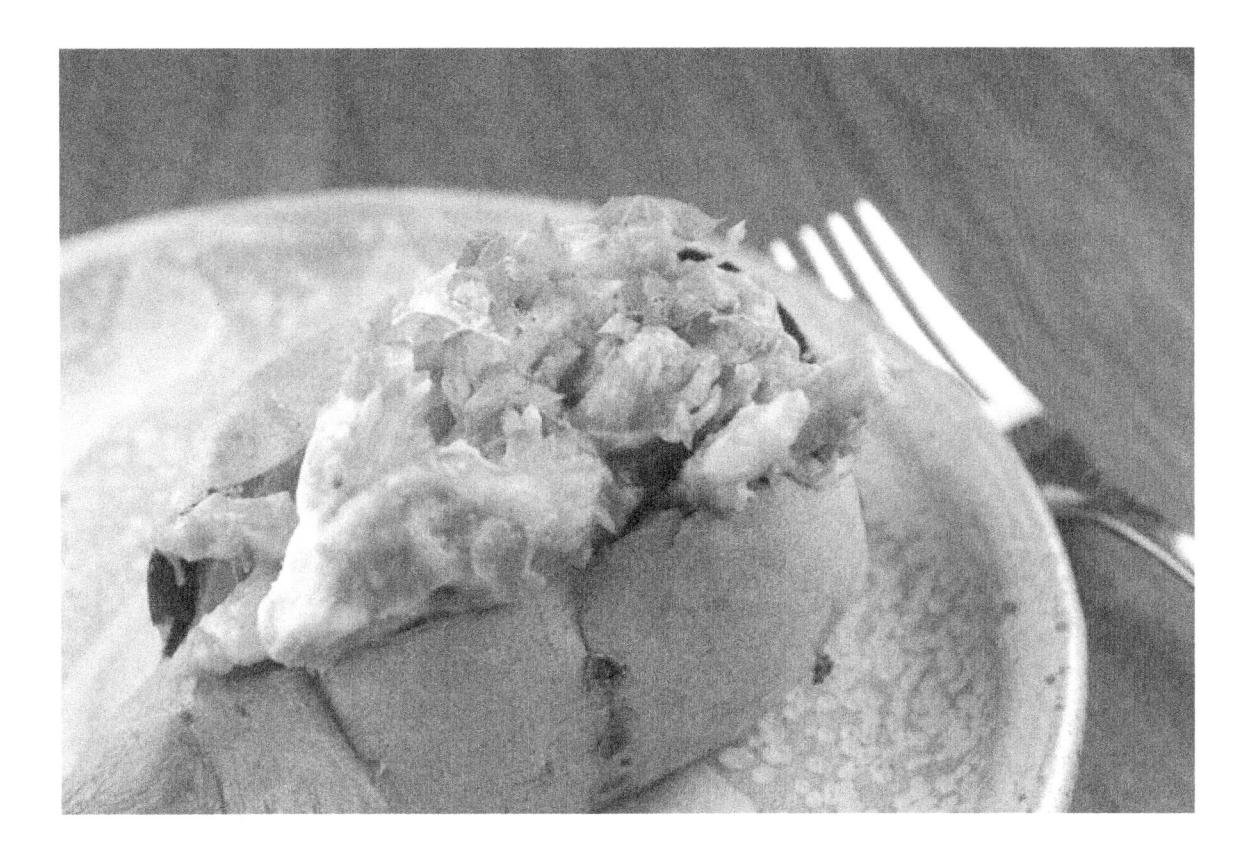

This may look like it takes a lot of time to prepare. But if you use cooked chicken (if you have leftovers from last night's dinner) and prepared curry sauce, it will only take you a few minutes of active preparation.

Serving Size: 4

Preparation Cooking Time: 30 minutes

Ingredients:

- 4 large sweet potatoes
- ½ cup curry sauce
- 8 oz. chicken, cooked and chopped
- 1 ½ cups cauliflower florets, steamed and chopped
- 4 teaspoons cilantro, chopped

Instructions:

1. Pierce the sweet potatoes using a fork.

2. Bake in the oven at 425 degrees F for 1 hour.

3. Place the sweet potatoes on a cutting board.

4. Slice lengthwise without cutting all the way through.

5. Pinch to expose the flesh.

6. Drizzle the sweet potatoes with the curry sauce.

7. Top with the chicken, cauliflower and cilantro.

8. Serve immediately.

Nutrients per Serving:

- Calories 257
- Fat 5.4 g
- Saturated fat 0.7 g
- Carbohydrates 29.5 g
- Fiber 5.3 g
- Protein 21.7 g
- Cholesterol 48 mg
- Sugars 11 g
- Sodium 240 mg
- Potassium 754 mg

Roasted Mushrooms

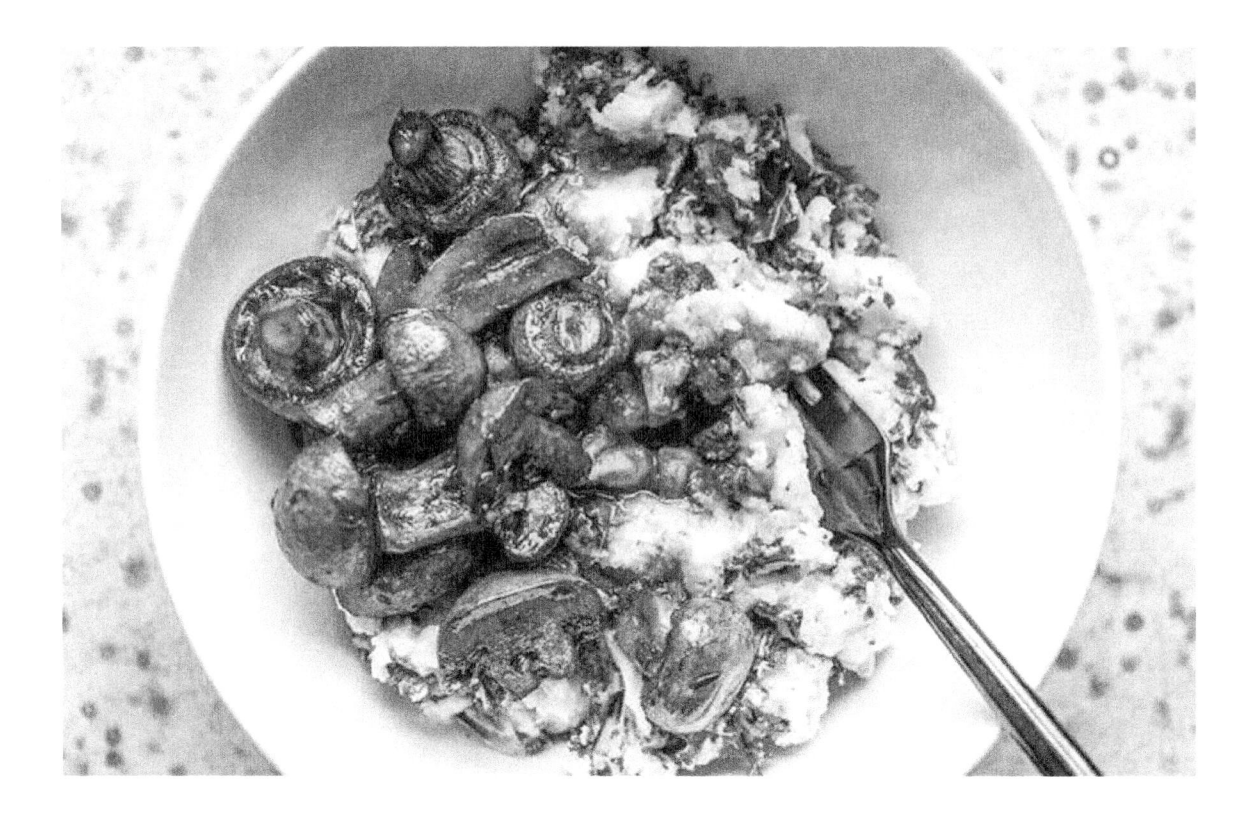

This simple and easy-to-prepare recipe helps you create mushrooms that have savory meaty flavors you surely can't get enough.

Serving Size: 4

Preparation Cooking Time: 30 minutes

Ingredients:

- 1 lb. mixed mushrooms
- 2 cups shallots, chopped
- 2 tablespoons olive oil
- Salt and pepper to taste
- 1 teaspoon dried thyme
- ¼ cup red wine

Instructions:

1. Preheat your oven to 450 degrees F.

2. Toss the mushrooms in the oil.

3. Season with the salt, pepper and thyme.

4. Transfer to a baking pan.

5. Roast in the oven for 15 minutes.

6. Stir in the red wine.

7. Roast for another 5 minutes.

Nutrients per Serving:

- Calories 178
- Fat 7.3 g
- Saturated fat 1 g
- Carbohydrates 20.6 g
- Fiber 3.6 g
- Protein 5.2 g
- Cholesterol 12 mg
- Sugars 10 g
- Sodium 163 mg
- Potassium 720 mg

Seared Tuna with Salad

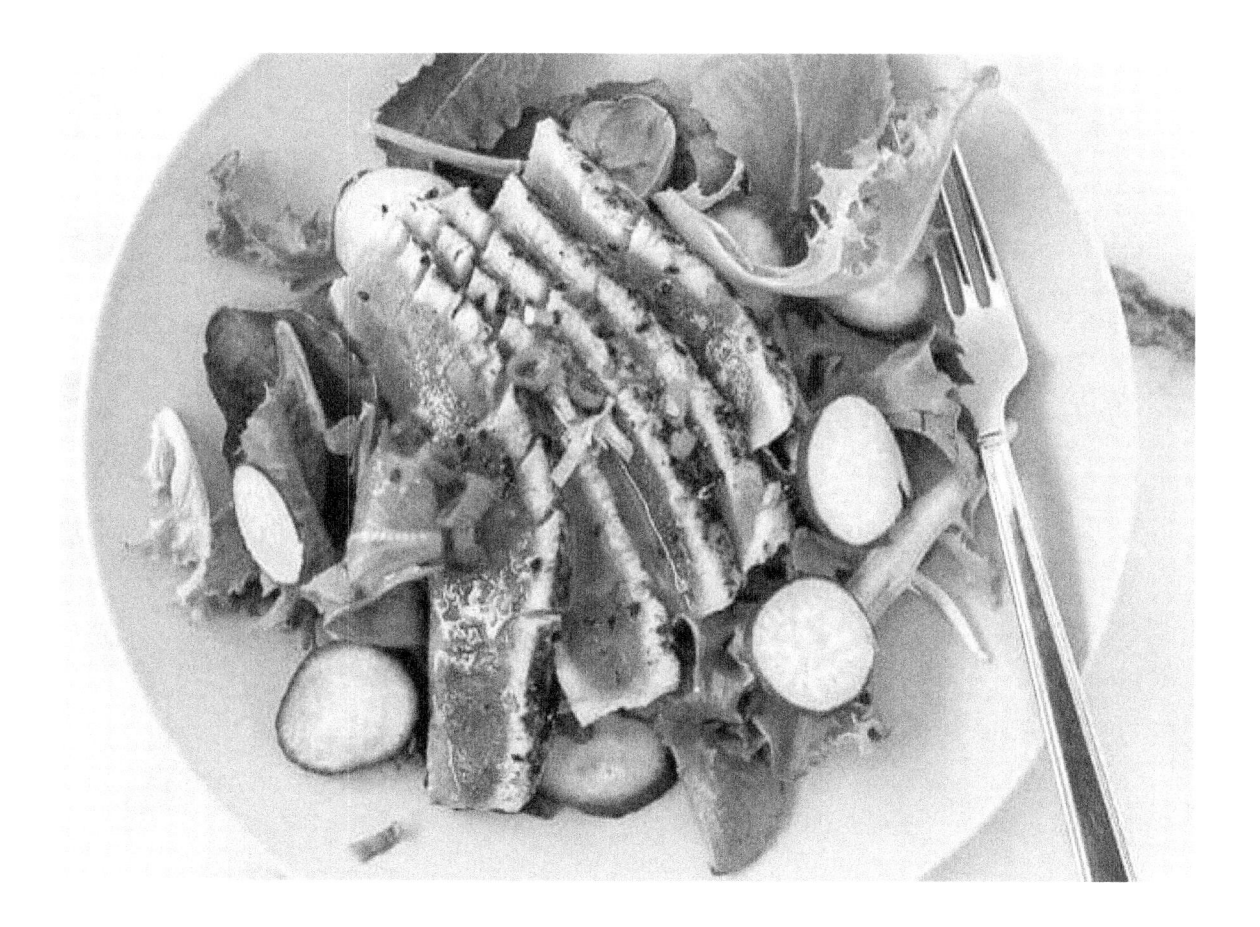

Tuna is a healthier alternative to red meat. In this recipe, we up the ante of plain tuna with fresh herbs, olive oil, lemon juice, bulgur, and chickpeas.

Serving Size: 4

Preparation Cooking Time: 45 minutes

Ingredients:

- 2 cups boiling water
- ½ cup bulgur
- ¼ cup olive oil, divided
- ½ cup lemon juice, divided
- 4 teaspoons freshly grated lemon zest, divided
- Salt and pepper to taste
- ¼ cup fresh Italian parsley, chopped
- ¼ cup fresh mint leaves, chopped
- 15 oz. chickpeas (unsalted)
- 4 tuna steaks
- 1 onion, sliced thinly
- ¼ cup fresh dill, chopped

Instructions:

1. Soak the bulgur in boiling water for 30 minutes.

2. Drain and transfer to a bowl.

3. Stir in half of the oil and half of the lemon zest.

4. Season with the salt and pepper.

5. Stir in the parsley, mint and chickpeas. Set aside.

6. Pour the remaining oil into a pan over medium heat.

7. Sear the tuna for 2 minutes per side.

8. Drain on a plate lined with paper towel.

9. Add the onion to the pan and cook for 5 minutes.

10. Reduce heat.

11. Add the tuna steaks to the pan.

12. Cook for 3 minutes per side.

13. In a bowl, mix the dill with the remaining lemon juice.

14. Place the tuna on a serving plate.

15. Top with the onions and drizzle with the dill mixture.

16. Serve with the chickpeas salad on the side.

Nutrients per Serving:

- Calories 459
- Fat 16.2 g
- Saturated fat 2.4 g
- Carbohydrates 43.2 g
- Fiber 8.2 g
- Protein 35.9 g
- Cholesterol 44 mg
- Sugars 2 g
- Sodium 557 mg
- Potassium 881 mg

Shrimp Pesto

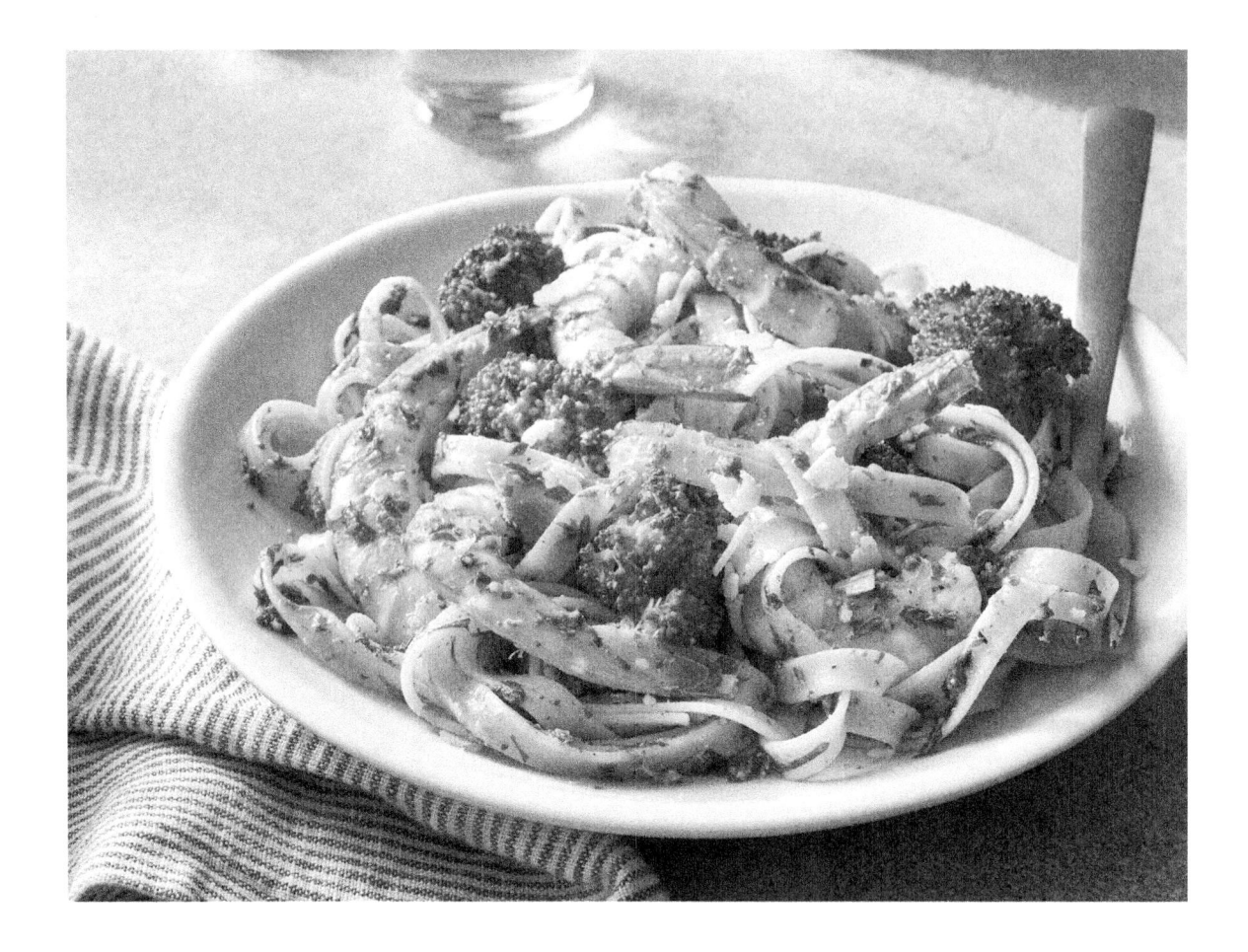

Here's a delicious way of preparing shrimp—flavor it up with pesto and add cherry tomatoes and avocado to the mix.

Serving Size: 4

Preparation Cooking Time: 25 minutes

Ingredients:

- ¼ cup pesto
- 1 tablespoon olive oil
- Salt and pepper to taste
- 2 tablespoons balsamic vinegar
- 1 lb. large shrimp, peeled and deveined
- 4 cups baby arugula
- 2 cups quinoa, cooked
- 1 avocado, sliced into small cubes
- 1 cup cherry tomatoes, sliced in half

Instructions:

1. In a bowl, mix the pesto, oil, salt, pepper and vinegar.

2. Take 4 tablespoons of this mixture and transfer to another bowl.

3. Set aside.

4. Cook the shrimp in a pan over medium heat for 5 minutes.

5. Transfer to a plate.

6. Add the quinoa and arugula to the first bowl.

7. Toss evenly with the sauce.

8. Top with the avocado, tomatoes and shrimp.

9. Drizzle with the remaining pesto mixture.

Nutrients per Serving:

- Calories 429
- Fat 22 g
- Saturated fat 3.6 g
- Carbohydrates 29.3 g
- Fiber 7.2 g
- Protein 30.9 g
- Cholesterol 188 mg
- Sugars 5 g
- Sodium 571 mg
- Potassium 901 mg

Provençal Fish Fillets

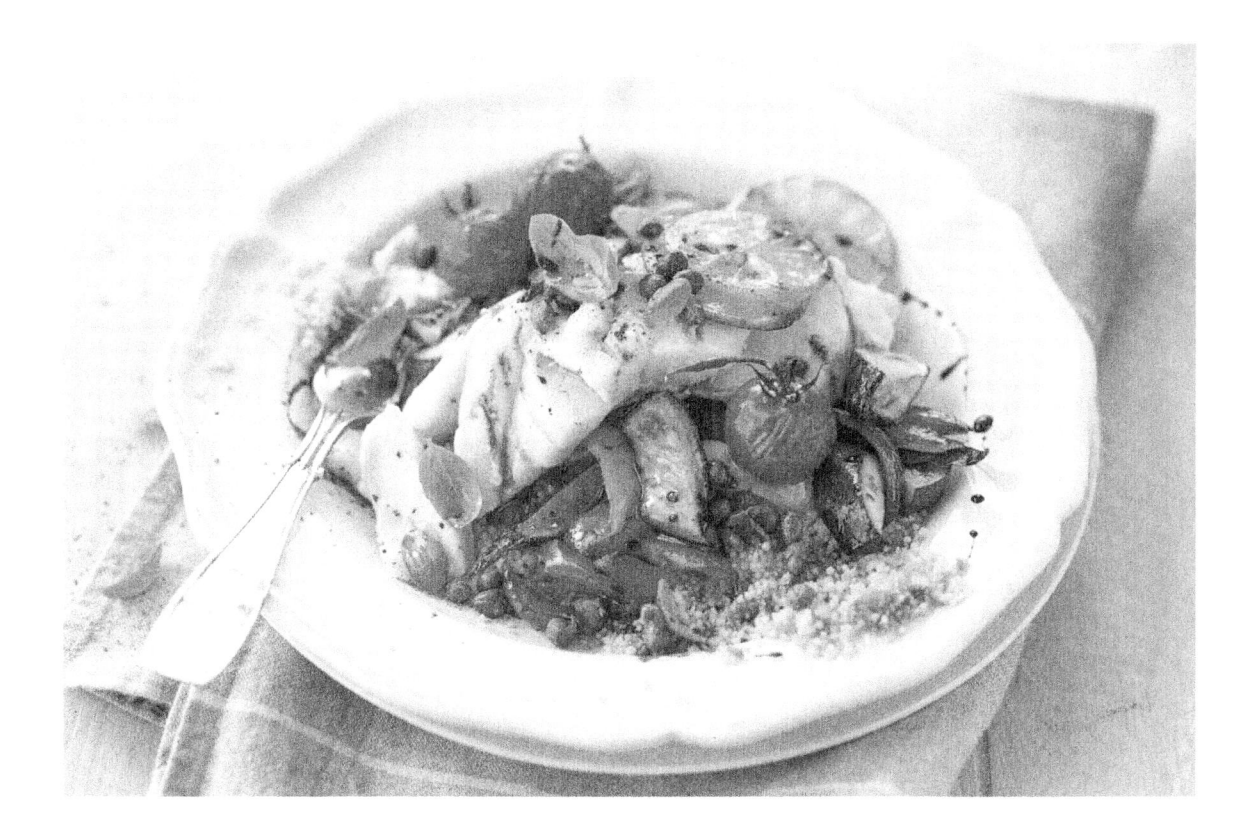

This fish fillet recipe is reminiscent of the flavors that popular in a region in France called Provence. Here, dishes are usually prepared by using onion, garlic, olive oil, olives, and tomatoes—the same ingredients used in this recipe.

Serving Size: 4

Preparation Cooking Time: 30 minutes

Ingredients:

- 4 cod fillets
- 1 tablespoon olive oil
- 1 onion sliced thinly
- 2 cloves garlic, crushed and minced
- 1 teaspoon capers, drained
- 8 olives, pitted and sliced in half
- 15 oz. canned whole tomatoes, drained and chopped
- 2 teaspoons fresh thyme leaves, chopped

Instructions:

1. Pour the oil into a pan over medium heat.

2. Cook the onion and garlic for 5 minutes, stirring frequently.

3. Stir in the capers, olives, tomatoes and thyme.

4. Simmer for 10 minutes.

5. Preheat your broiler.

6. Broil the fish for 5 minutes per side.

7. Serve with the sauce.

Nutrients per Serving:

- Calories 161
- Fat 5.2 g
- Saturated fat 0.8 g
- Carbohydrates 7.2 g
- Fiber 1.6 g
- Protein 21.4 g
- Cholesterol 48 mg
- Sugars 4 g
- Sodium 292 mg
- Potassium 700 mg

Crunchy Salmon Fillet

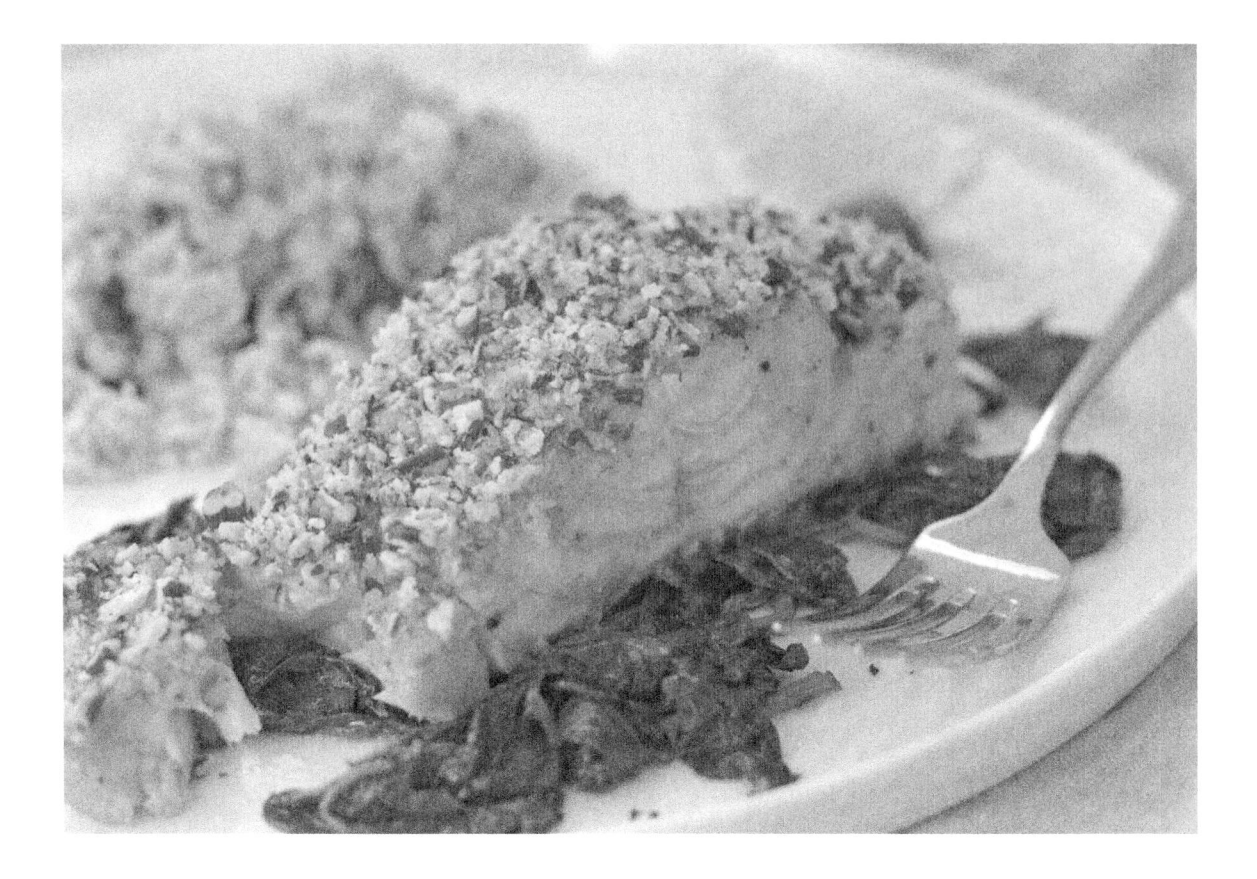

Ditch the regular breading and opt for pumpkin seeds, which produce a crunchy texture for your salmon.

Serving Size: 4

Preparation Cooking Time: 40 minutes

Ingredients:

- 1 lb. carrots, sliced
- ¼ cup pure maple syrup, divided
- ½ teaspoon pumpkin pie spice
- Salt to taste
- 3 tablespoons roasted pumpkin seeds, chopped
- 8 saltine crackers, crushed
- 4 salmon fillets
- Cooking spray

Instructions:

1. Preheat your oven to 425 degrees F.

2. Line your baking pan with foil.

3. Add the carrots to a bowl.

4. Toss in half of maple syrup, pumpkin pie spice and salt.

5. Transfer to the baking pan.

6. Bake in the oven for 10 minutes. Set aside.

7. In another bowl, combine the pumpkin seeds and crushed crackers.

8. Sprinkle with a little salt.

9. Brush both sides of the fish with the remaining maple syrup.

10. Sprinkle both sides with the cracker mixture and press to adhere.

11. Spray both sides with oil.

12. Bake for 15 minutes.

13. Serve the salmon with the carrots.

Nutrients per Serving:

- Calories 359
- Fat 14.6 g
- Saturated fat 2.3 g
- Carbohydrates 30.6 g
- Fiber 4.1 g
- Protein 27.9 g
- Cholesterol 62 mg
- Sugars 19 g
- Sodium 519 mg
- Potassium 1064 mg

Pot Roast

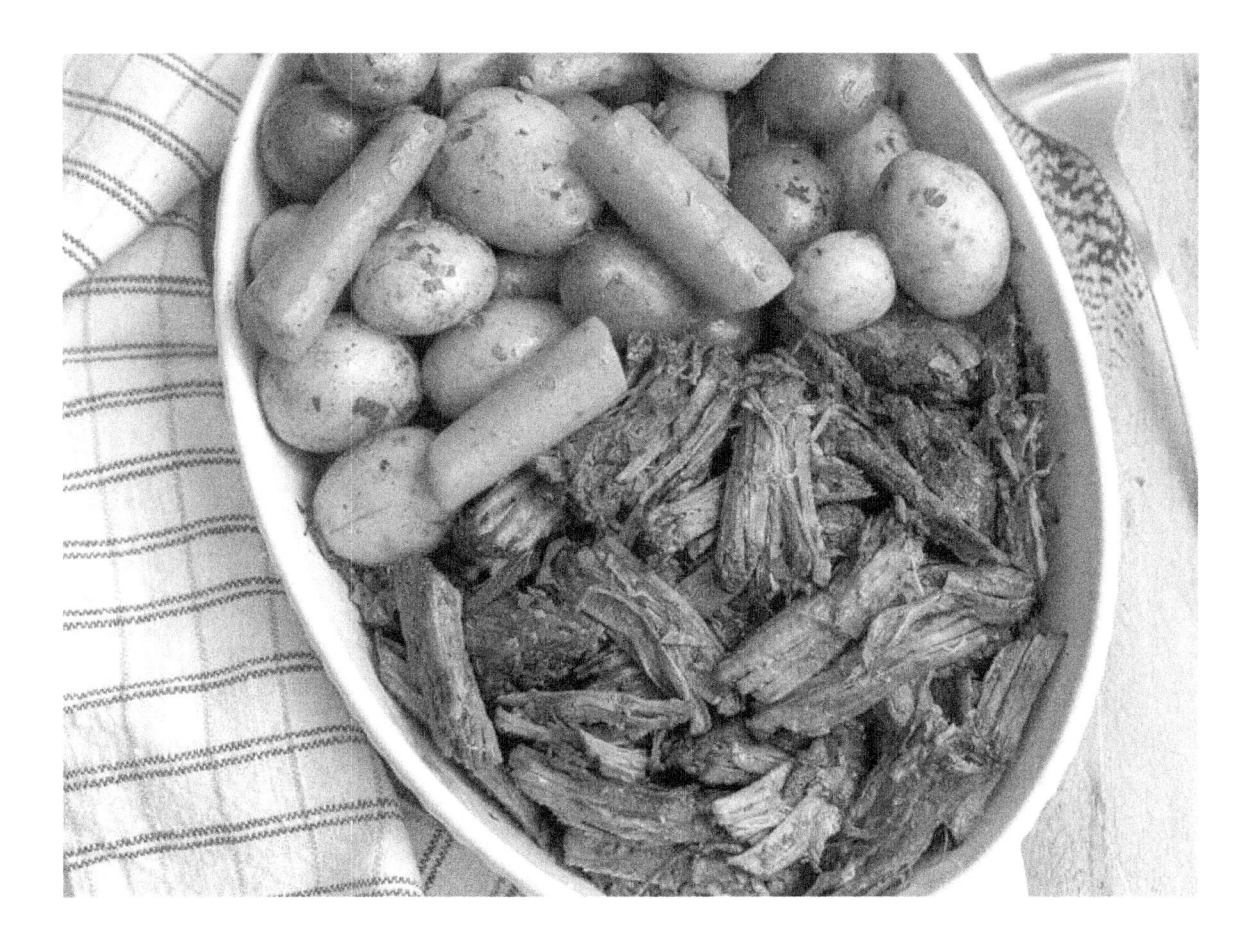

Who said you couldn't have pot roast again? Here's a healthy version of this dish that you can prepare anytime you're craving for it.

Serving Size: 8

Preparation Cooking Time: 5 hours and 15 minutes

Ingredients:

- 3 lb. boneless beef chuck pot roast, fat trimmed
- 2 teaspoons garlic pepper seasoning
- ½ cup water
- 1 tablespoons canned chipotle peppers in adobo sauce
- 7 oz. mixed dried fruits
- 1 tablespoon cold water
- 2 teaspoons cornstarch
- 4 cups cooked mashed potatoes

Instructions:

1. Season all sides of the roast with the garlic pepper.

2. Add to your slow cooker.

3. Pour in the water, chipotle peppers and dried fruits.

4. Cover the pot.

5. Cook on high for 5 hours.

6. Place the roast and fruits on a plate.

7. Pour the cooking liquid to a bowl and remove the fat.

8. Add the remaining cooking liquid to a pan.

9. Mix 1 tablespoon water and cornstarch.

10. Add this to the pan as well.

11. Cook while stirring for 2 minutes.

12. Slice the roast.

13. Drizzle the gravy on top.

14. Serve with the dried fruits and mashed potatoes.

Nutrients per Serving:

- Calories 338
- Fat 6.7 g
- Saturated fat 2.5 g
- Carbohydrates 36.1 g
- Fiber 2.4 g
- Protein 34 g
- Cholesterol 94 mg
- Sugars 2 g
- Sodium 436 mg
- Potassium 986 mg

Curry Fish

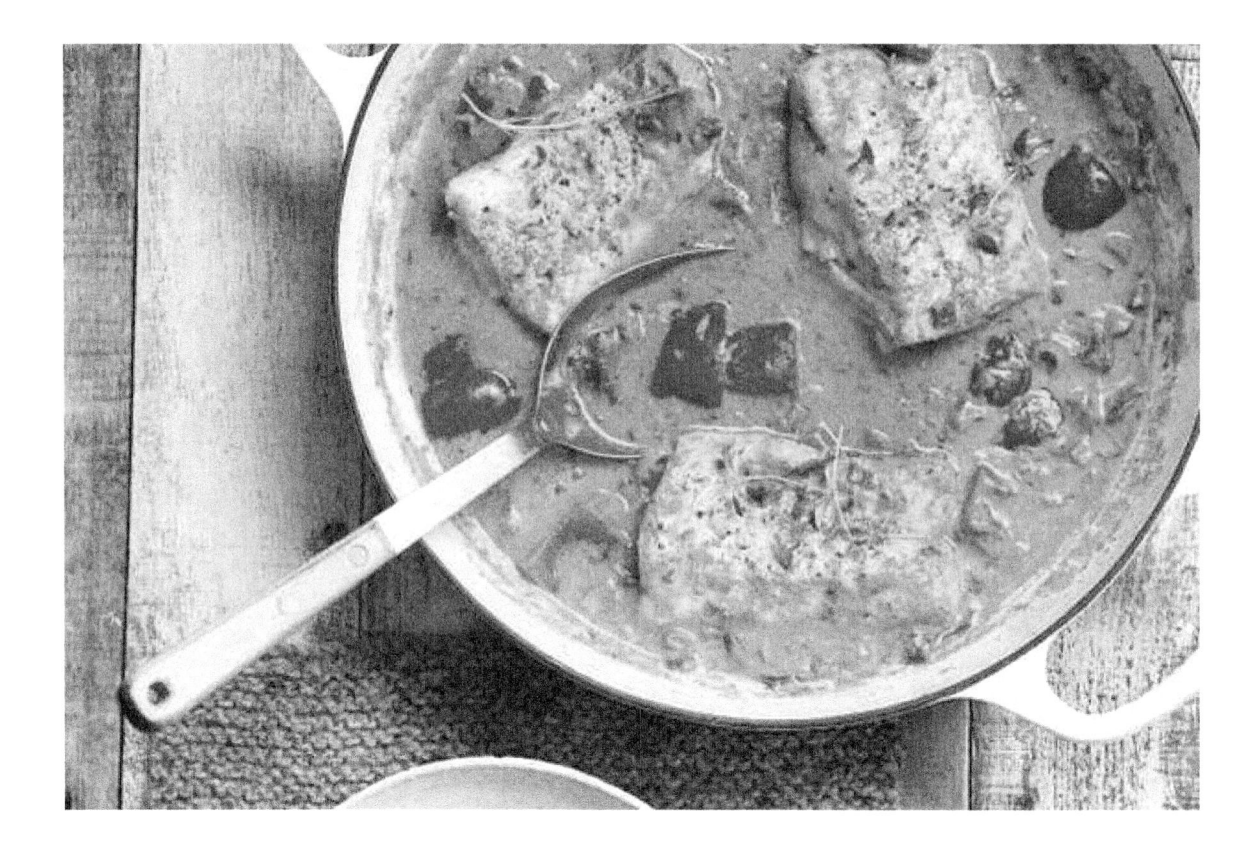

Bake your seasoned fish fillet and serve with lentils and cherry tomatoes for a quick, light, and delicious dinner meal.

Serving Size: 4

Preparation Cooking Time: 30 minutes

Ingredients:

- 4 white fish fillets
- Salt and pepper to taste
- 1 tablespoon olive oil
- 2 cups cherry tomatoes, sliced in half
- 2 cups fresh pea pods
- ½ teaspoon garam masala, divided
- 1 teaspoon curry powder, divided
- 1 tablespoon fresh cilantro leaves, chopped and divided
- 1 ⅓ cups cooked lentils

Instructions:

1. Preheat your oven to 450 degrees F.

2. Season the fish with the salt and pepper.

3. Add the fish on a baking pan.

4. Bake for 6 to 7 minutes or until fish is flaky.

5. Transfer to a plate.

6. Pour the olive oil into a pan over medium heat.

7. Cook the tomatoes and pea pods for 3 minutes.

8. Season with half of the garam masala, half of the curry powder and half of the cilantro.

9. Add the remaining garam masala, curry powder and cilantro to the cooked lentils.

10. Serve the fish with the tomato mixture and the cooked lentils.

Nutrients per Serving:

- Calories 283
- Fat 6.3 g
- Saturated fat 1.6 g
- Carbohydrates 22 g
- Fiber 7.9 g
- Protein 36.6 g
- Cholesterol 71 mg
- Sugars 5 g
- Sodium 231 mg
- Potassium 903 mg

Salmon Salad

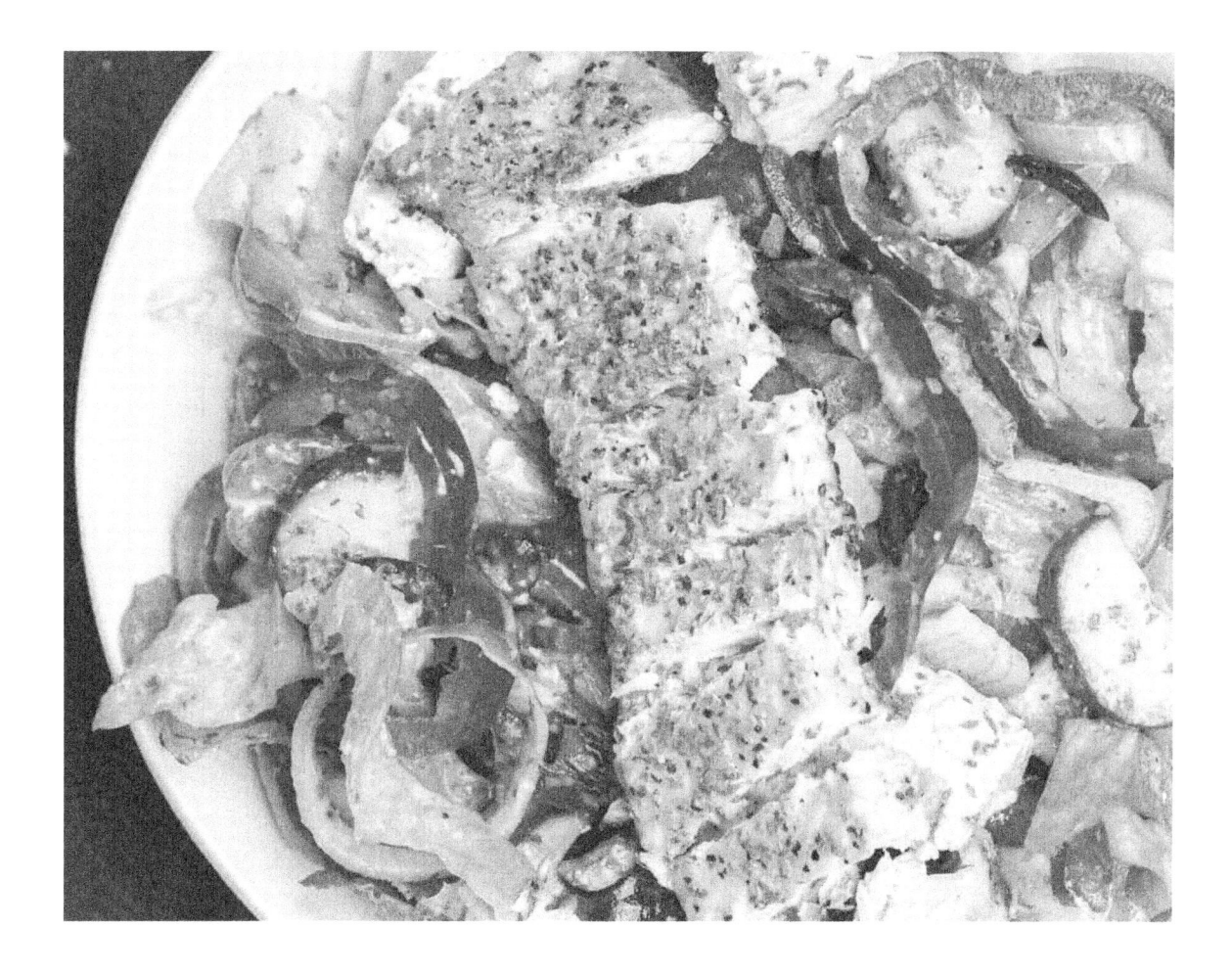

You've probably tried many versions of salmon salad before. But this one makes by using grilled salmon. So, you can expect something different and exciting.

Serving Size: 4

Preparation Cooking Time: 1 hour

Ingredients:

- 1 tablespoon powdered fruit pectin
- 1 teaspoon fresh dill weed, chopped
- ¼ cup water
- Pepper to taste
- 1 teaspoon Dijon honey mustard
- 2 teaspoons white-wine vinegar
- 4 salmon fillets
- 3 cups mixed greens, chopped
- 1 cup steamed green beans, sliced
- 1 cup cucumber, sliced
- ½ cup radish, sliced
- ¼ cup scallions, chopped

Instructions:

1. Prepare the dressing my mixing the powdered fruit pectin, fresh dill weed, water, pepper, Dijon honey mustard and white-wine vinegar.

2. Chill in the refrigerator for 30 minutes.

3. Season the salmon with the pepper.

4. Grill the salmon for 5 minutes per side.

5. In a bowl, mix the remaining ingredients.

6. Transfer the salad on 4 serving plates.

7. Top with the grilled salmon, and drizzle with the mustard mixture.

Nutrients per Serving:

- Calories 228
- Fat 9.1 g
- Saturated fat 1.4 g
- Carbohydrates 5.4 g
- Fiber 2 g
- Protein 30 g
- Cholesterol 78 mg
- Sugars 2 g
- Sodium 83 mg
- Potassium 981 mg

Garlic Shrimp with Spinach

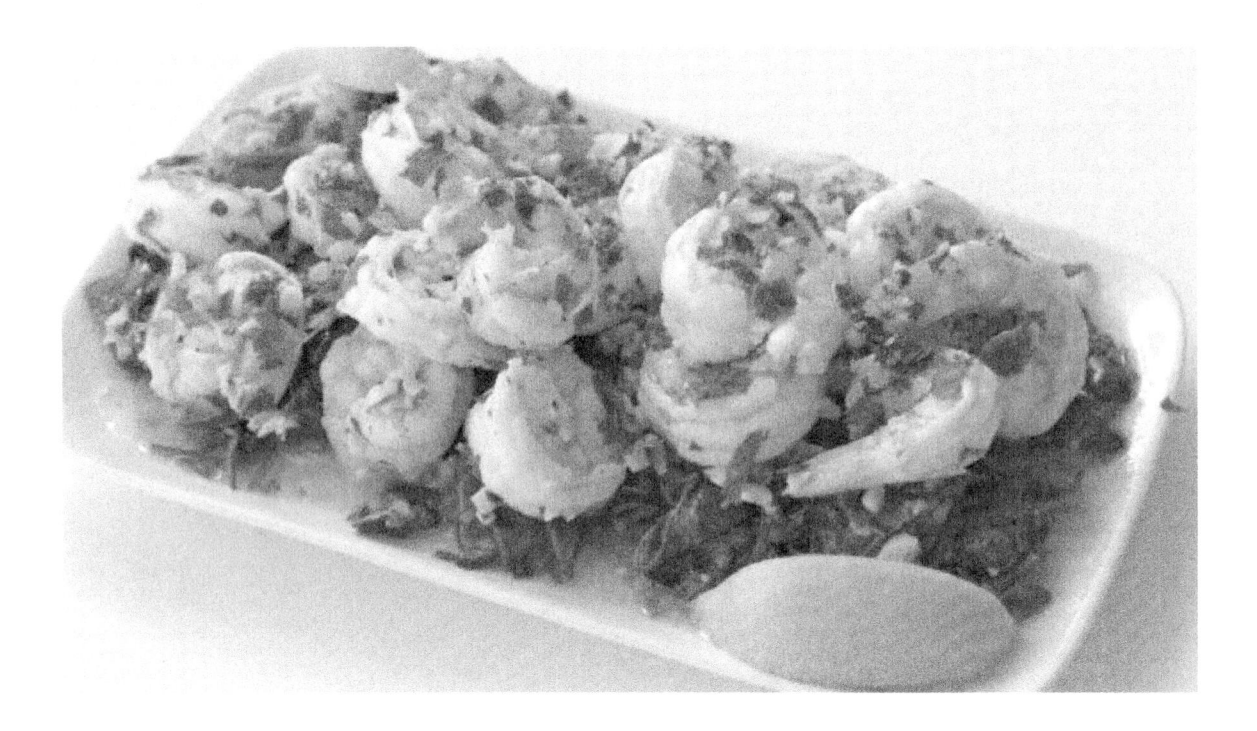

You'll love this version of garlic shrimp, and you'd probably add this to your weekly menu rotation.

Serving Size: 4

Preparation Cooking Time: 30 minutes

Ingredients:

- 6 cloves garlic, sliced and divided
- 3 tablespoons olive oil, divided
- 1 lb. spinach
- Salt and pepper to taste
- 1 tablespoon freshly squeezed lemon juice
- 1 lb. shrimp, peeled and deveined
- 1 tablespoon fresh parsley, chopped
- 1 ½ teaspoons freshly grated lemon zest
- ¼ teaspoon red pepper flakes

Instructions:

1. Pour 1 tablespoon olive oil into a pot over medium high heat.

2. Cook half of the garlic for 1 minute, stirring frequently.

3. Reduce heat and add the spinach.

4. Season with the salt.

5. Cook for 2 minutes.

6. Stir in the lemon juice.

7. Remove from heat and transfer to a serving plate.

8. Pour the remaining oil to the pot.

9. Cook the remaining garlic for 2 minutes.

10. Add the shrimp and red pepper flakes and season with the salt.

11. Cook for 5 minutes.

12. Top the spinach with the shrimp.

13. Garnish with the parsley and lemon zest.

Nutrients per Serving:

- Calories 226
- Fat 11.6 g
- Saturated fat 1.7 g
- Carbohydrates 6.1 g
- Fiber 2.7 g
- Protein 26.4 g
- Cholesterol 183 mg
- Sugars 1 g
- Sodium 444 mg
- Potassium 963 mg

Salmon with Kale Creamy Dressing

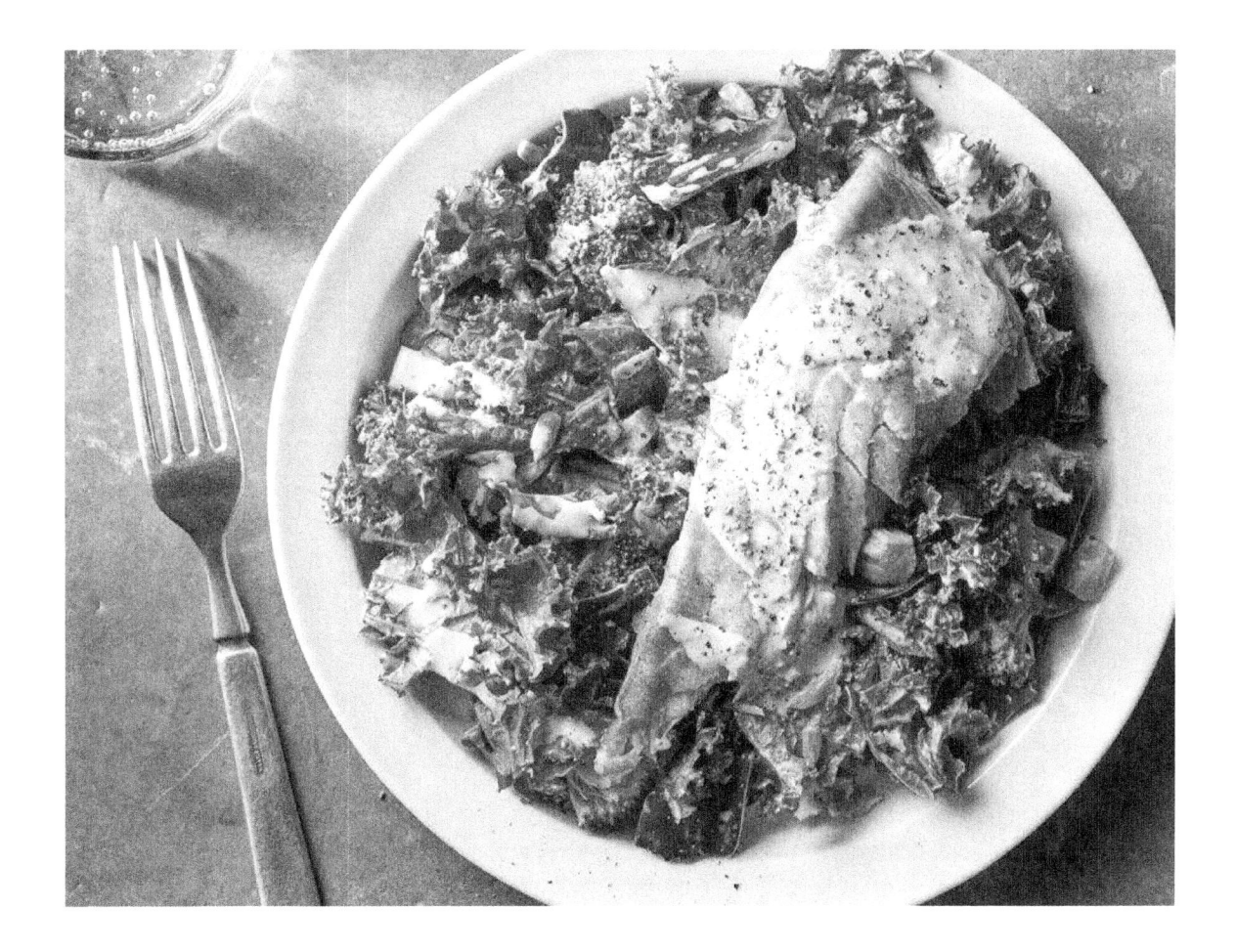

In this a quick and easy recipe, we serve salmon on the top of chopped kale and drizzle it with a delicious and creamy dressing.

Serving Size: 4

Preparation Cooking Time: 30 minutes

Ingredients:

- 4 salmon fillets
- ¼ cup light mayonnaise
- ½ cup reduced-fat plain yogurt
- 2 tablespoons freshly squeezed lemon juice
- 1 tablespoon fresh parsley leaves, chopped
- 1 tablespoon fresh chives, snipped
- 2 tablespoons freshly grated Parmesan cheese
- 2 teaspoons low-sodium soy sauce
- Pepper to taste
- 1 clove garlic, crushed and minced
- 2 cups broccoli, steamed and chopped
- 8 cups curly kale, chopped
- 2 cups carrots, diced
- 2 cups red cabbage, chopped
- ½ cup sunflower seeds, toasted

Instructions:

1. Preheat your broiler.

2. Line your baking pan with foil.

3. Add the salmon on the baking pan.

4. Broil for 10 minutes, flipping once.

5. In a bowl, mix the mayo, yogurt, lemon juice, parsley, chives, soy sauce, pepper and garlic.

6. In another bowl, combine the remaining ingredients.

7. Transfer the salad on serving plates.

8. Top each one with the salmon.

9. Drizzle with the dressing.

Nutrients per Serving:

- Calories 409
- Saturated fat 24.2 g
- Carbohydrates 4.2 g
- Fiber 5.8 g
- Protein 31.9 g
- Cholesterol 63 mg
- Sugars 7 g
- Sodium 356 mg
- Potassium 1152 mg

Herbed Scallops with Asparagus

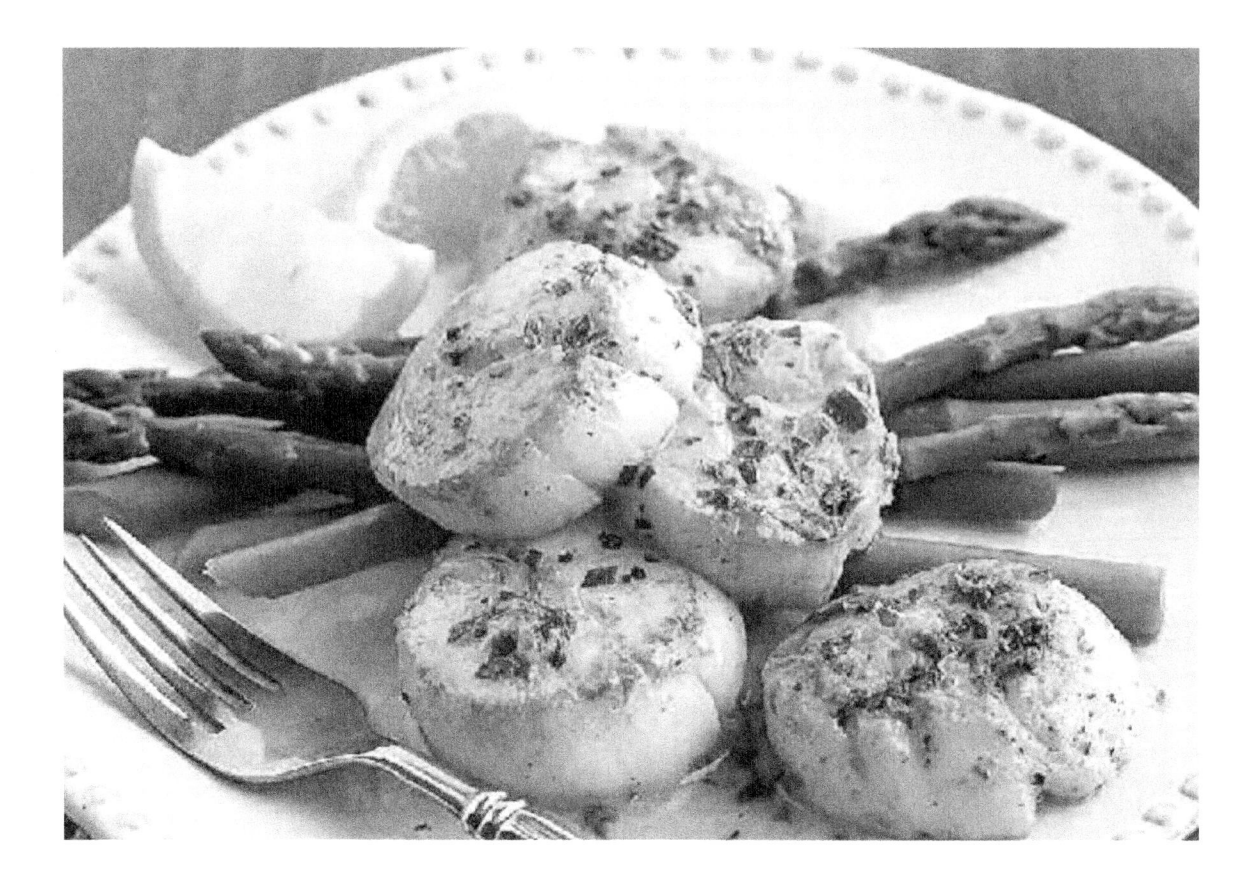

This is a great way to enjoy seafood—prepare a delicious meal without having to stress yourself out. Try this recipe—herbed scallop with butter and asparagus.

Serving Size: 4

Preparation Cooking Time: 15 minutes

Ingredients:

- 1 ¼ lb. scallops
- Salt and pepper to taste
- 1 tablespoon olive oil
- 1 lb. asparagus spears, trimmed and steamed
- 3 tablespoons vegetable oil spread
- 1 tablespoons lemon juice
- 1 teaspoon lemon zest
- 1 tablespoon fresh tarragon, chopped
- 1 lemon, sliced into wedges

Instructions:

1. Season the scallops with the salt and pepper.

2. Add the oil to a pan over medium heat.

3. Cook the scallops for 3 minutes.

4. Flip and cook for another 2 minutes.

5. Place the steamed asparagus on a plate.

6. Top with the scallops.

7. Add the oil spread, lemon juice, lemon zest and tarragon to a pan.

8. Cook for 1 minute.

9. Drizzle the mixture over the scallops and asparagus.

10. Garnish with the lemon wedges.

Nutrients per Serving:

- Calories 253
- Fat 11.9 g
- Saturated fat 2.4 g
- Carbohydrates 13.8 g
- Fiber 5 g
- Protein 27 g
- Cholesterol 47 mg
- Sugars 3 g
- Sodium 436 mg
- Potassium 773 mg

Zucchini Noodles with Meat Veggies

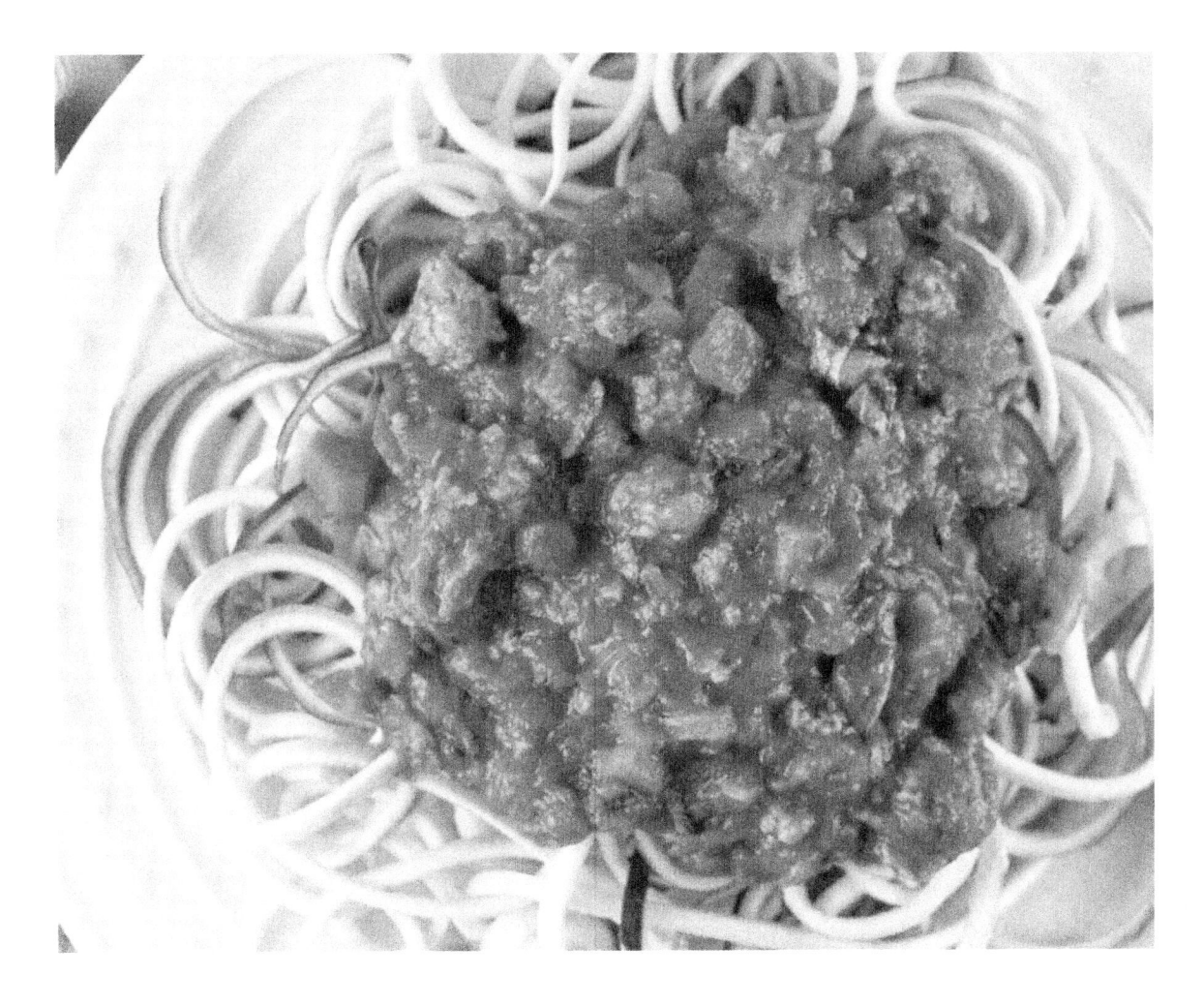

There are many ways to prepare zucchini noodles. Here's one that you will definitely enjoy—zucchini noodles topped with meat, vegetables, and cheese.

Serving Size: 6

Preparation Cooking Time: 1 hour

Ingredients:

- 1 tablespoon olive oil
- ½ cup onion, chopped
- 2 cloves garlic, crushed and minced
- ½ cup celery, chopped
- ½ cup carrot, chopped
- 8 oz. lean ground beef
- 14 oz. canned diced tomatoes with herbs (unsalted)
- 8 oz. tomato sauce (unsalted)
- ¼ cup water
- Salt and pepper to taste
- ¼ teaspoon red pepper flakes
- 1 teaspoon dried Italian seasoning
- 2 zucchinis, sliced into very thin strands
- 8 oz. mushrooms, sliced
- 3 tablespoons Parmesan cheese, grated

Instructions:

1. Add the oil to a pan over medium heat.

2. Cook the onion, garlic, celery, carrot and ground beef for 3 to 5 minutes.

3. Drain the oil.

4. Stir in the diced tomatoes, tomato sauce, water, salt, pepper, red pepper flakes and Italian seasoning.

5. Bring to a boil.

6. Reduce heat and simmer for 10 minutes.

7. Spray a larger pan with oil.

8. Put this over medium high heat.

9. Cook the mushrooms for 5 minutes.

10. Add the zucchini and cook for 2 minutes.

11. Drain the mixture.

12. Transfer the zucchini noodles with mushrooms on a serving plate.

13. Pour the meat sauce on top.

14. Sprinkle with the Parmesan cheese before serving.

Nutrients per Serving:

- Calories 158
- Fat 4.6 g
- Saturated fat 1.8 g
- Carbohydrates 17.8 g
- Fiber 8.5 g
- Protein 12.5 g
- Cholesterol 26 mg
- Sugars 12 g
- Sodium 334 mg
- Potassium 769 mg

Turkey Salad

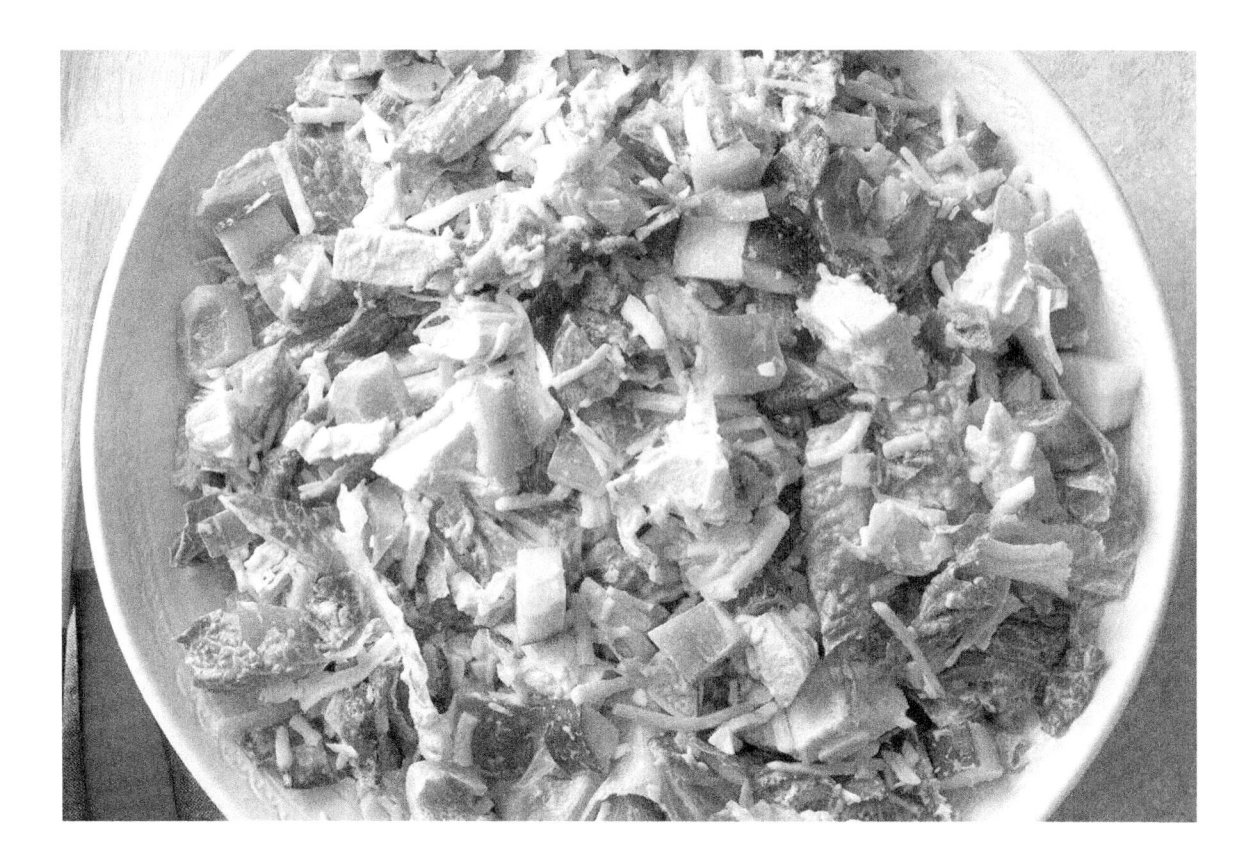

Do you have leftover turkey from last night's dinner? Transform it into something incredible by shredding the turkey and serving it with the top of crunchy Romaine lettuce along with corn kernels and strips of tortilla and bell pepper.

Serving Size: 4

Preparation Cooking Time: 40 minutes

Ingredients:

- 1 teaspoon poppy seeds
- 1 tablespoon olive oil
- 1 tablespoon freshly squeezed lime juice
- ¼ cup freshly squeezed orange juice
- 1 tablespoon honey
- 1 teaspoon olive oil
- 2 cups corn kernels
- 6 cups Romaine lettuce, chopped
- 2 cups cooked turkey, chopped or shredded
- ¼ cup onion, chopped
- 1 orange bell pepper, sliced into strips
- 1 cup tomatoes, chopped
- 2 slices cooked crisp, turkey bacon, and crumbled
- 2 corn tortillas, sliced into strips and toasted

Instructions:

1. Prepare the dressing by mixing the poppy seeds, olive oil, lime juice, orange juice and honey. Set aside.

2. Preheat your oven to 350 degrees F.

3. Pour the olive oil into a pan over medium heat.

4. Cook the corn kernels for 7 minutes.

5. In a bowl, combine the rest of the ingredients except the tortilla strips.

6. Drizzle the salad with the poppy seed mixture, and top with the tortilla strips.

Nutrients per Serving:

- Calories 334
- Fat 8.4 g
- Saturated fat 1.5 g
- Carbohydrates 35.6 g
- Fiber 5.3 g
- Protein 32.2 g
- Cholesterol 76 mg
- Sugars 11 g
- Sodium 188 mg
- Potassium 846 mg

Rosemary Turkey Roast

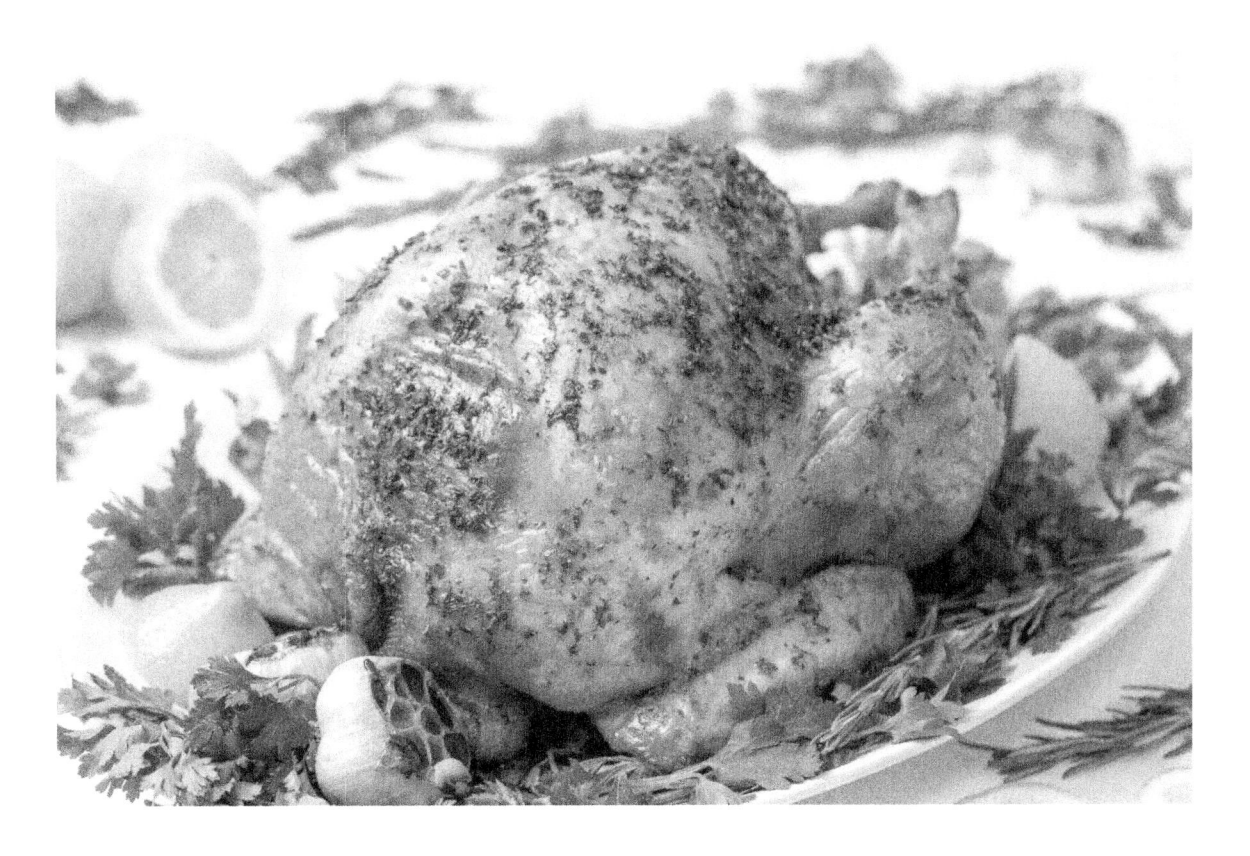

Season turkey breast with rosemary, drizzle it with gravy, and serve with vegetables to create a simple yet tasty dinner for the family.

Serving Size: 8

Preparation Cooking Time: 5 hours

Ingredients:

- Salt and pepper to taste
- ¼ teaspoon garlic powder
- ¼ teaspoon dried thyme, crushed
- 1 teaspoon dried rosemary, crushed
- 1 tablespoon vegetable oil
- 3 lb. turkey breast fillet
- Cooking spray
- 1 onion, sliced into wedges
- 8 carrots, sliced
- 1 lb. baby potatoes, sliced in half
- ¼ cup low-sodium chicken broth
- ¼ cup all-purpose flour

Instructions:

1. In a bowl, mix the salt, pepper, garlic powder, thyme and rosemary.

2. Season both sides of the turkey breast with this mixture.

3. Pour the oil in a pan over medium heat.

4. Cook the turkey until brown on both sides.

5. Spray your slow cooker with oil.

6. Add the onion, carrots and potatoes in your slow cooker.

7. Top with the turkey.

8. Cover the pot.

9. Cook on low for 4 hours and 30 minutes.

10. Transfer the turkey and veggies on a serving plate.

11. Strain the cooking liquid into a pan.

12. Combine the cooking liquid, flour and broth.

13. Simmer until thick.

14. Pour the sauce over the turkey and veggies before serving.

Nutrients per Serving:

- Calories 256
- Fat 2.7 g
- Saturated fat 0.5 g
- Carbohydrates 23.4 g
- Fiber 3.7 g
- Protein 33.5 g
- Cholesterol 76 mg
- Sugars 5 g
- Sodium 272 mg
- Potassium 800 mg

Spaghetti Squash with Tomato Basil

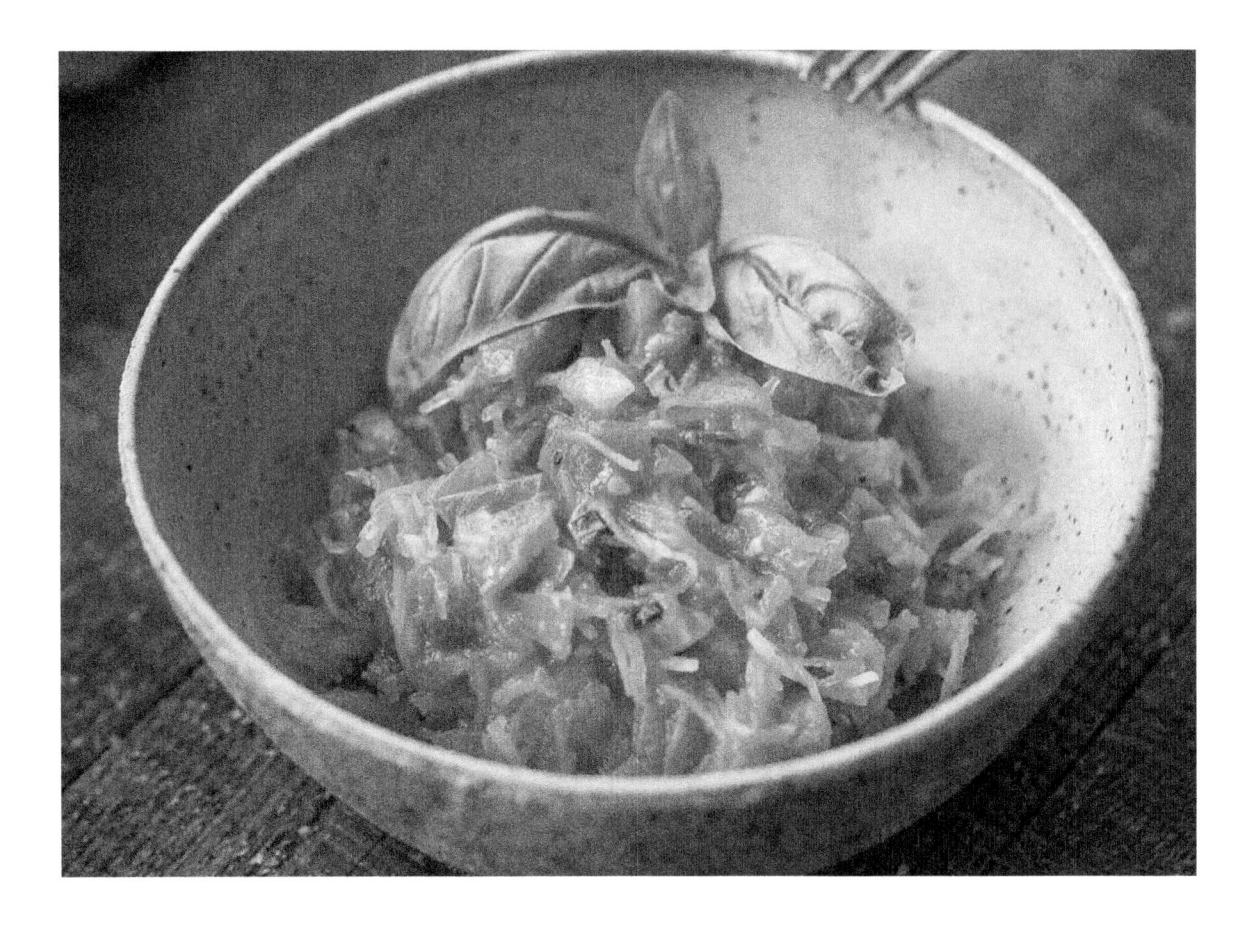

Replacing regular pasta with spaghetti squash. It is a sure way to reduce calories and carbs in this quick and delicious dinner recipe.

Serving Size: 4

Preparation Cooking Time: 1 hour

Ingredients:

- 3 tablespoons olive oil
- 1 onion, chopped
- 4 cloves garlic, crushed and minced
- 4 cups tomatoes, diced
- ¼ cup dry red wine
- Salt and pepper to taste
- 10 basil leaves, chopped
- 4 cups cooked spaghetti squash

Instructions:

1. Add the oil to a pan over medium heat.

2. Cook the onion for 3 minutes.

3. Reduce heat and add the garlic.

4. Cook for 2 minutes.

5. Add the tomatoes and red wine. Cook for 4 minutes.

6. Season with the salt and pepper.

7. Stir in the basil and spaghetti squash. Serve immediately.

Nutrients per Serving:

- Calories 268
- Fat 12 g
- Saturated fat 1.8 g
- Carbohydrates 37.2 g
- Fiber 8.5 g
- Protein 4.9 g
- Cholesterol 13 mg
- Sugars 17 g
- Sodium 322 mg
- Potassium 1028 mg

Mushroom Wrap

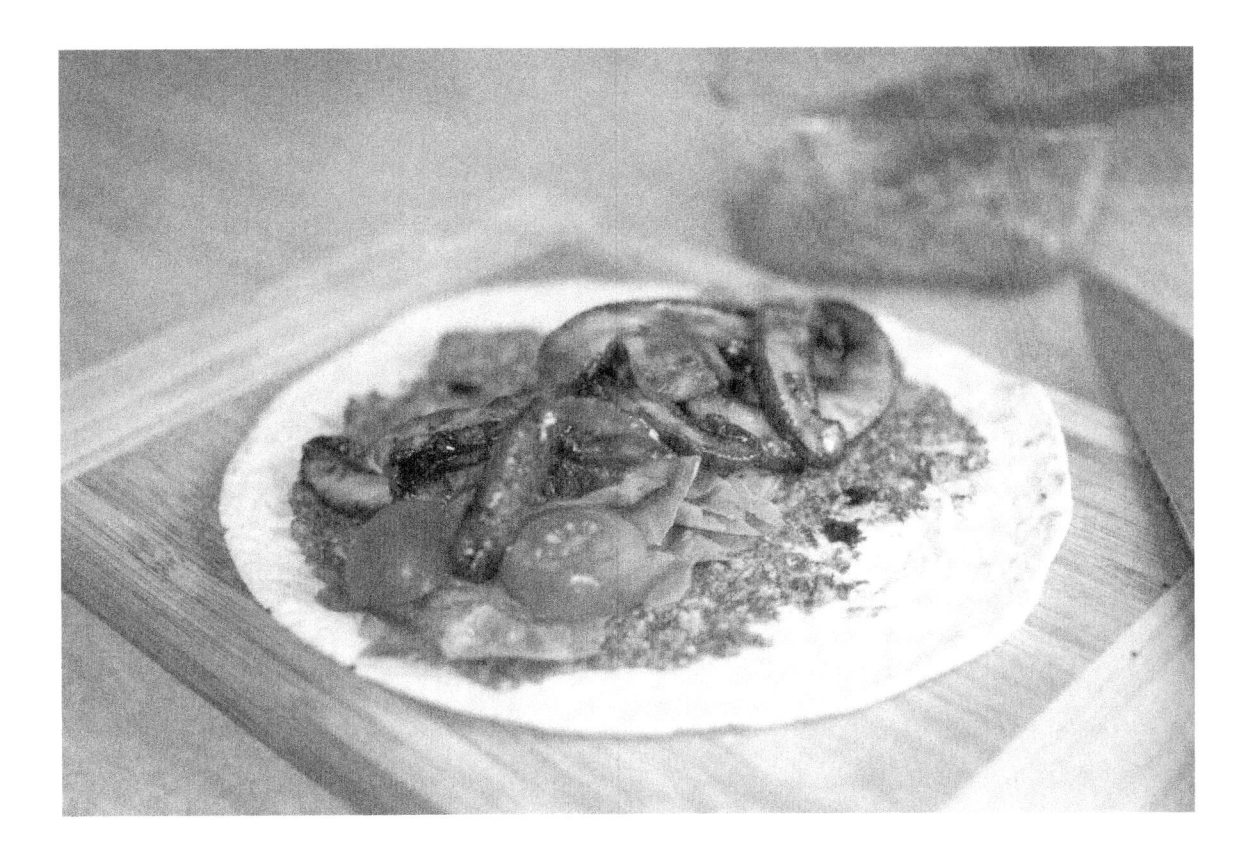

This is one meatless wrap that you're sure to enjoy, even if you're not a vegetarian! Find out how to prepare this quick snack.

Serving Size: 4

Preparation Cooking Time: 2 hours and 30 minutes

Ingredients:

- 4 mushrooms, gills and stems removed
- ¼ cup low-fat Italian salad dressing
- 4 whole-wheat wraps
- 1 yellow bell pepper
- 2 tablespoons basil pesto
- 1 tomato, sliced
- 8 lettuce leaves
- Cooking spray

Instructions:

1. Place the mushrooms caps in a bowl.

2. Pour in the salad dressing.

3. Toss to coat evenly.

4. Cover with foil and marinate in the refrigerator for 2 hours.

5. Spray the peppers with oil.

6. Grill the mushrooms and peppers for 7 minutes.

7. Place the wraps on your kitchen table.

8. Spread each one with the pesto.

9. Divide the tomatoes and lettuce among the wraps.

10. Top with the peppers and mushrooms.

11. Roll up the wraps and serve.

Nutrients per Serving:

- Calories 257
- Fat 10.5 g
- Saturated fat 2 g
- Carbohydrates 28.1 g
- Fiber 14 g
- Protein 13.3 g
- Cholesterol 3 mg
- Sugars 7 g
- Sodium 563 mg
- Potassium 817 mg

Chicken Salad with Avocado Pineapple

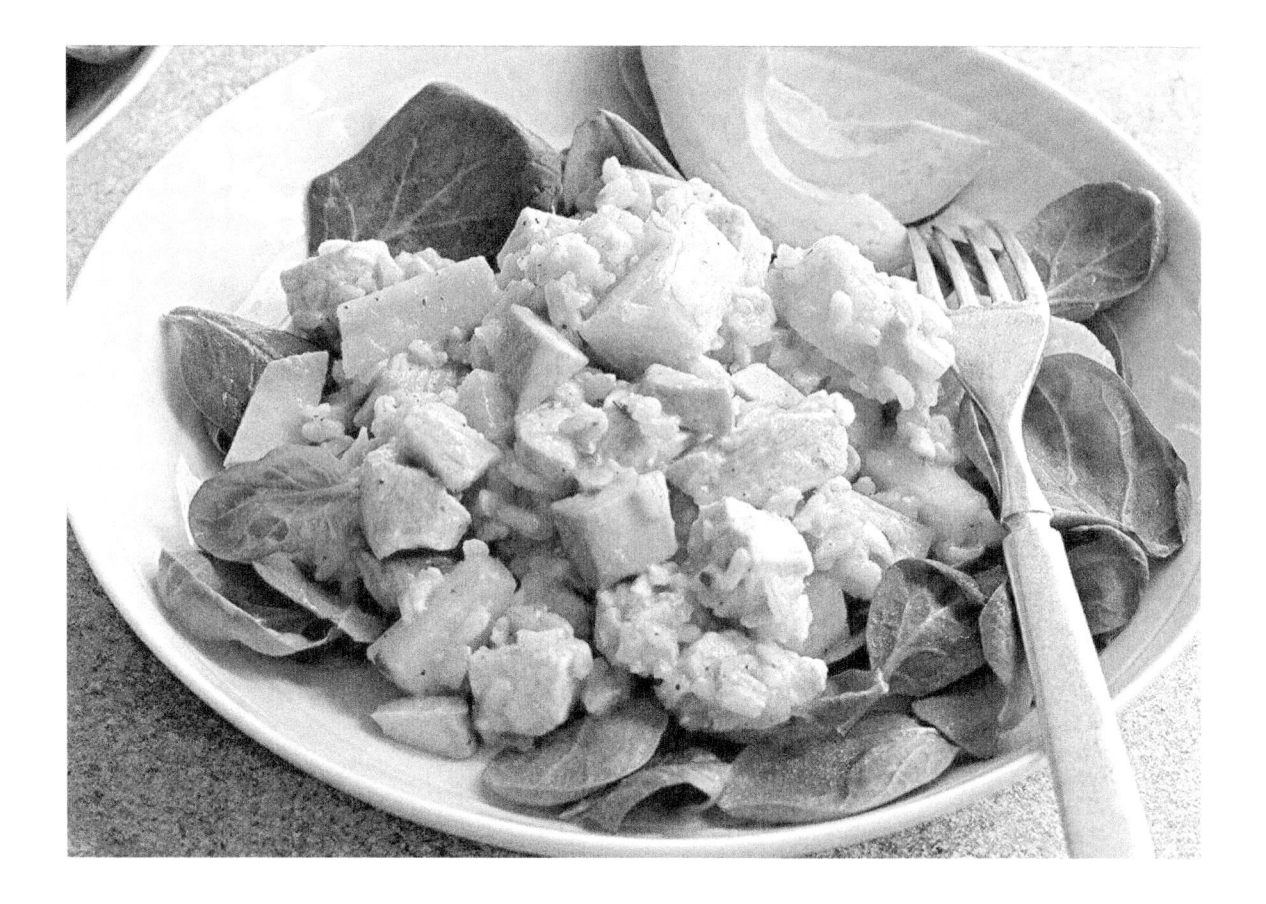

Have fun with creating this simple but flavorful chicken salad recipe. But what's even more exciting is when you eat it with your family and friends and enjoy this light and healthy meal together.

Serving Size: 4

Preparation Cooking Time: 30 minutes

Ingredients:

- 5 teaspoons vegetable oil, divided
- 5 tablespoons freshly squeezed lime juice, divided
- ⅛ teaspoon red pepper flakes
- 2 cloves garlic, crushed and minced
- 1 lb. chicken breast fillet, chopped
- Cooking spray
- Salt and pepper to taste
- ½ teaspoon ground ginger
- 1 teaspoon sugar
- 2 cups cooked brown rice
- 1 avocado, sliced in half and peeled
- 4 cups spinach, shredded
- 2 cups canned pineapple chunks, drained

Instructions:

1. Add 2 teaspoons oil, 1 tablespoon lime juice, red pepper flakes and garlic in a bowl.

2. Mix well.

3. Coat the chicken with this mixture.

4. Spray your pan with oil.

5. Place the pan over medium high heat.

6. Add the chicken with its marinade in the pan.

7. Cook for 7 minutes.

8. Transfer to a plate.

9. In another bowl, combine the remaining oil and lime juice with the salt, pepper, ginger and sugar.

10. Stir in the brown rice, avocado, spinach and pineapple chunks.

11. Top with the chicken.

Nutrients per Serving:

- Calories 421
- Fat 15 g
- Saturated fat 2.1 g
- Carbohydrates 42.5 g
- Fiber 5.8 g
- Protein 30.1 g
- Cholesterol 83 mg
- Sugars 9 g
- Sodium 372 mg
- Potassium 906 mg

Beef Burgundy with Mashed Potatoes

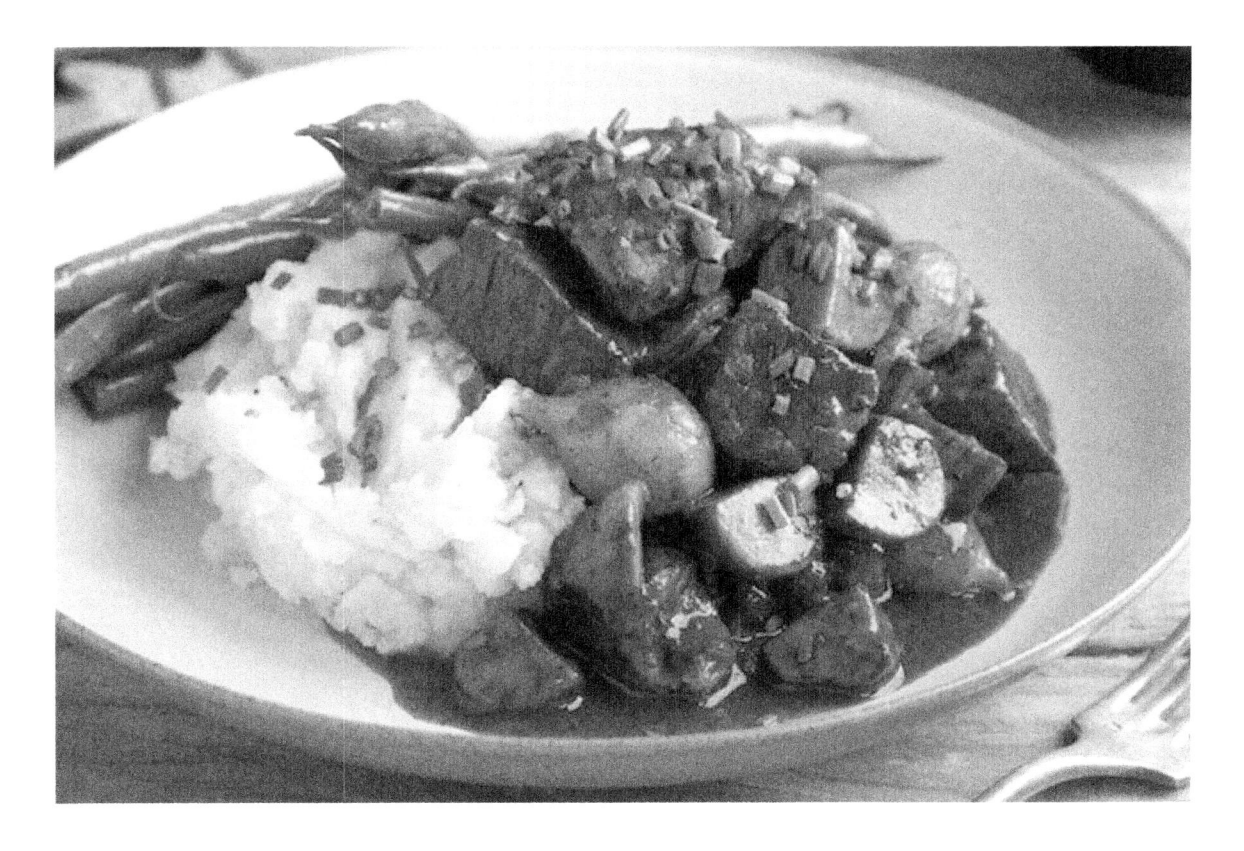

This dish is typically served with noodles, but for this recipe, we opt to pair it with garlic mashed potatoes, and the result is so amazing.

Serving Size: 8

Preparation Cooking Time: 5 hours

Ingredients:

- 4 teaspoons olive oil, divided
- 2 lb. beef chuck pot roast, sliced into cubes
- 3 onions, chopped
- 2 cups frozen onions
- 1 tablespoon butter
- 2 cloves garlic, crushed and minced
- 4 carrots, sliced
- 2 tablespoons quick-cooking tapioca
- ½ cup reduced-sodium beef broth
- 1 tablespoon tomato paste
- 1 cup Burgundy wine
- ¼ cup brandy
- Pepper to taste
- ½ teaspoon dried rosemary, crushed
- 2 bay leaves
- 1 cup mushrooms, sliced
- Mashed potatoes
- 1 lb. potatoes, sliced into wedges
- 4 cloves garlic, peeled and sliced
- Salt and pepper to taste
- 4 tablespoons nonfat milk
- 1 teaspoon dried thyme, crushed

Instructions:

1. Add half of the oil in a pan over medium heat.

2. Brown the beef on both sides.

3. Add the onions, frozen onions, garlic, and carrots in your slow cooker.

4. Sprinkle the tapioca on top.

5. Add the beef on top of the veggies.

6. In a bowl, mix the beef broth, tomato paste, wine, brandy, pepper, dried rosemary, and dried thyme.

7. Pour this mixture into the slow cooker.

8. Stir in the bay leaves.

9. Cover the pot and cook on high for 4 hours.

10. Remove the bay leaves.

11. In a pot filled with water, boil the potatoes with the garlic for 25 minutes.

12. Mash the potatoes with a fork or potato masher.

13. Stir in the butter.

14. Season with the pepper and salt.

15. Beat in the milk until potatoes are fluffy.

16. Cook the mushrooms in the remaining oil until brown.

17. Add these to the beef mixture.

18. Serve the beef with the mashed potatoes.

Nutrients per Serving:

- Calories 344
- Fat 8.8 g
- Saturated fat 3.1 g
- Carbohydrates 28 g
- Fiber 3.8 g
- Protein 28.7 g
- Cholesterol 78 mg
- Sugars 6 g
- Sodium 255 mg
- Potassium 1059 mg

Tofu Soup with Veggies

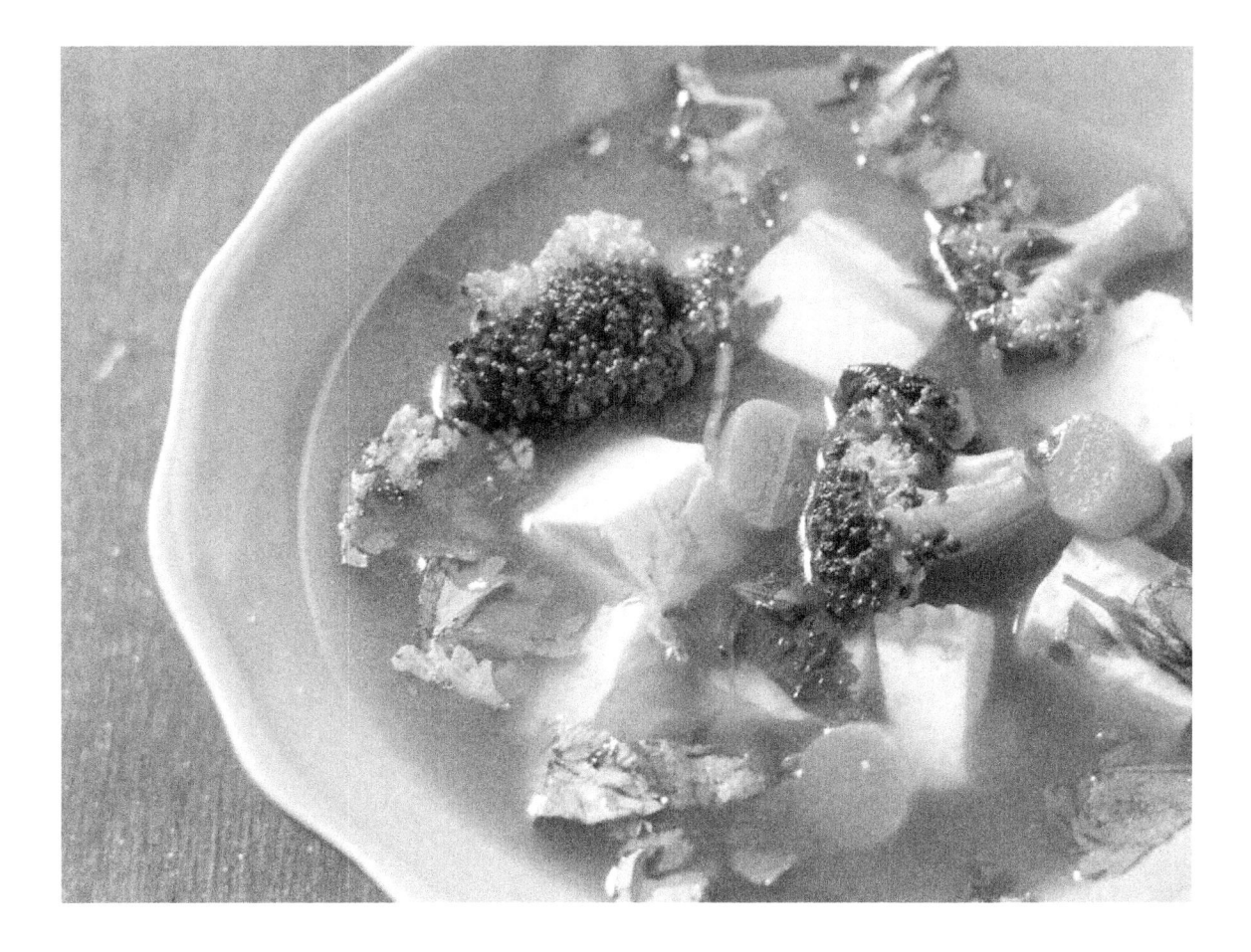

If you're looking for a comforting soup recipe that doesn't take a lot of effort to prepare, try this tofu soup with vegetables. You can replace the vegetables with whatever you have available in your pantry.

Serving Size: 4

Preparation Cooking Time: 2 hours and 40 minutes

Ingredients:

- 12 oz. tofu, sliced into cubes
- 2 tablespoons olive oil
- 1 teaspoon dried Italian seasoning, crushed
- Cooking spray
- 15 oz. canned diced tomatoes with herbs
- 2 cups chicken broth
- ½ cup asparagus, sliced
- ½ cup peas
- 8 oz. mushrooms, sliced
- ¼ cup green olives, sliced
- ½ cup roasted red sweet pepper, chopped
- ¼ cup dried tomatoes packed in oil, drained and chopped

Instructions:

1. Add the tofu in a bowl.

2. Coat with oil and sprinkle with the Italian seasoning.

3. Cover the bowl and marinate in the refrigerator for 2 hours.

4. Spray your pan with oil.

5. Put it over medium high heat.

6. Cook the tofu for 3 to 4 minutes per side.

7. Pour in the tomatoes and broth.

8. Bring to a boil.

9. Add the asparagus, mushrooms and peas.

10. Simmer for 6 minutes.

11. Stir in the rest of the ingredients.

12. Serve warm.

Nutrients per Serving:

- Calories 259
- Fat 14.9 g
- Saturated fat 1.8 g
- Carbohydrates 19.2 g
- Fiber 9.8 g
- Protein 15.6 g
- Cholesterol 13 mg
- Sugars 11 g
- Sodium 574 mg
- Potassium 722 mg

Jerk Chicken

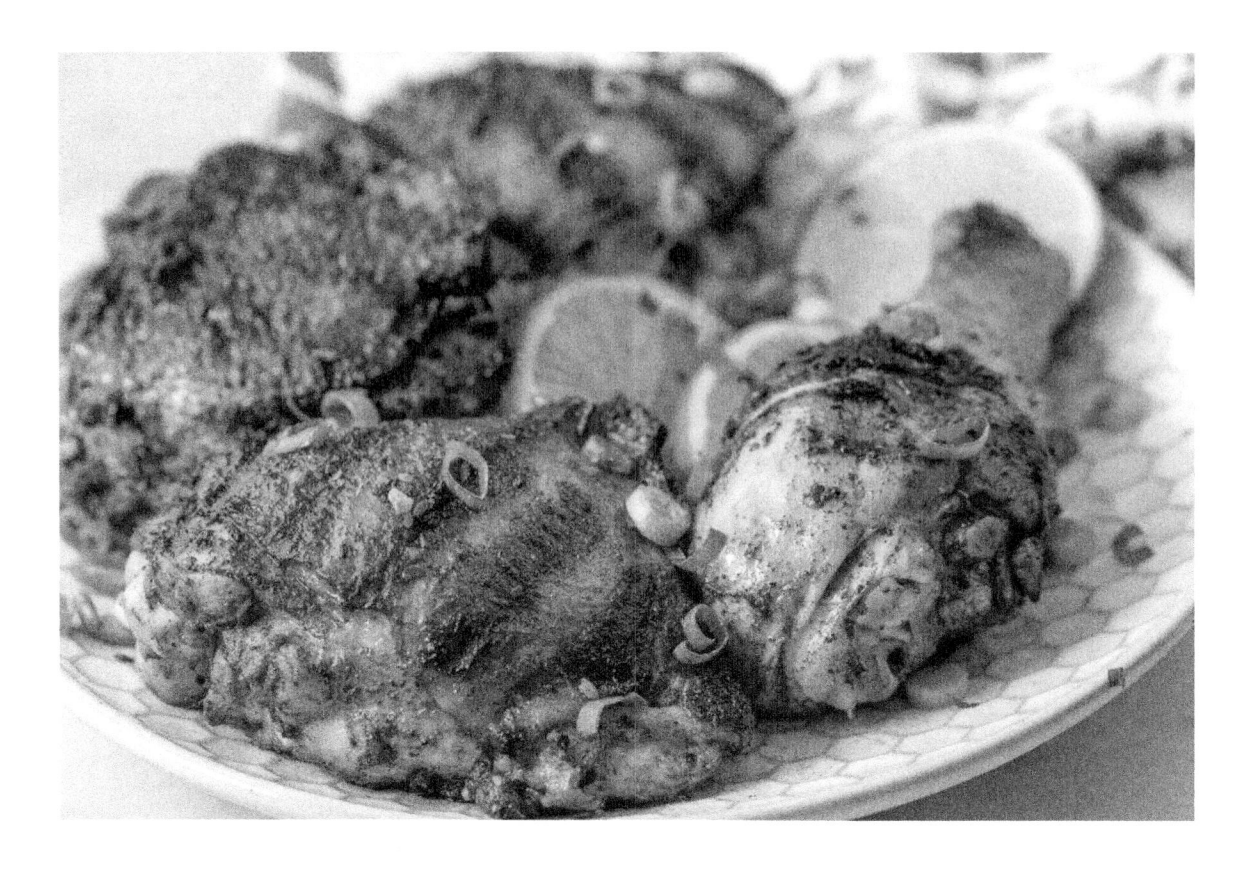

Consider this recipe when you're running out of time but want to create a delicious meal for the family. This is jerk chicken served with pineapple slaw.

Serving Size: 4

Preparation Cooking Time: 30 minutes

Ingredients:

- 1 cup pineapple chunks
- 2 cups red cabbage, shredded
- 3 heads bok choy, sliced
- 4 teaspoons brown sugar, divided
- 2 tablespoons cider vinegar
- 2 teaspoons all-purpose flour
- 2 teaspoons jerk seasoning
- 4 chicken breast fillets

Instructions:

1. Combine the pineapple, red cabbage and bok choy in a bowl.

2. In a smaller bowl, mix 2 teaspoons brown sugar with the vinegar.

3. Pour the mixture over the pineapple mixture. Toss to coat evenly.

4. Add the remaining brown sugar, flour and seasoning in a bowl.

5. Coat the chicken with the mixture.

6. Cook the chicken over medium heat for 10 minutes, flipping once.

7. Serve the chicken with the pineapple slaw.

Nutrients per Serving:

- Calories 238
- Fat 6.6 g
- Saturated fat 0.9 g
- Carbohydrates 18.7 g
- Fiber 2.9 g
- Protein 26.9 g
- Cholesterol 72 mg
- Sugars 13 g
- Sodium 350 mg
- Potassium 819 mg

Steak with Mushroom Sauce

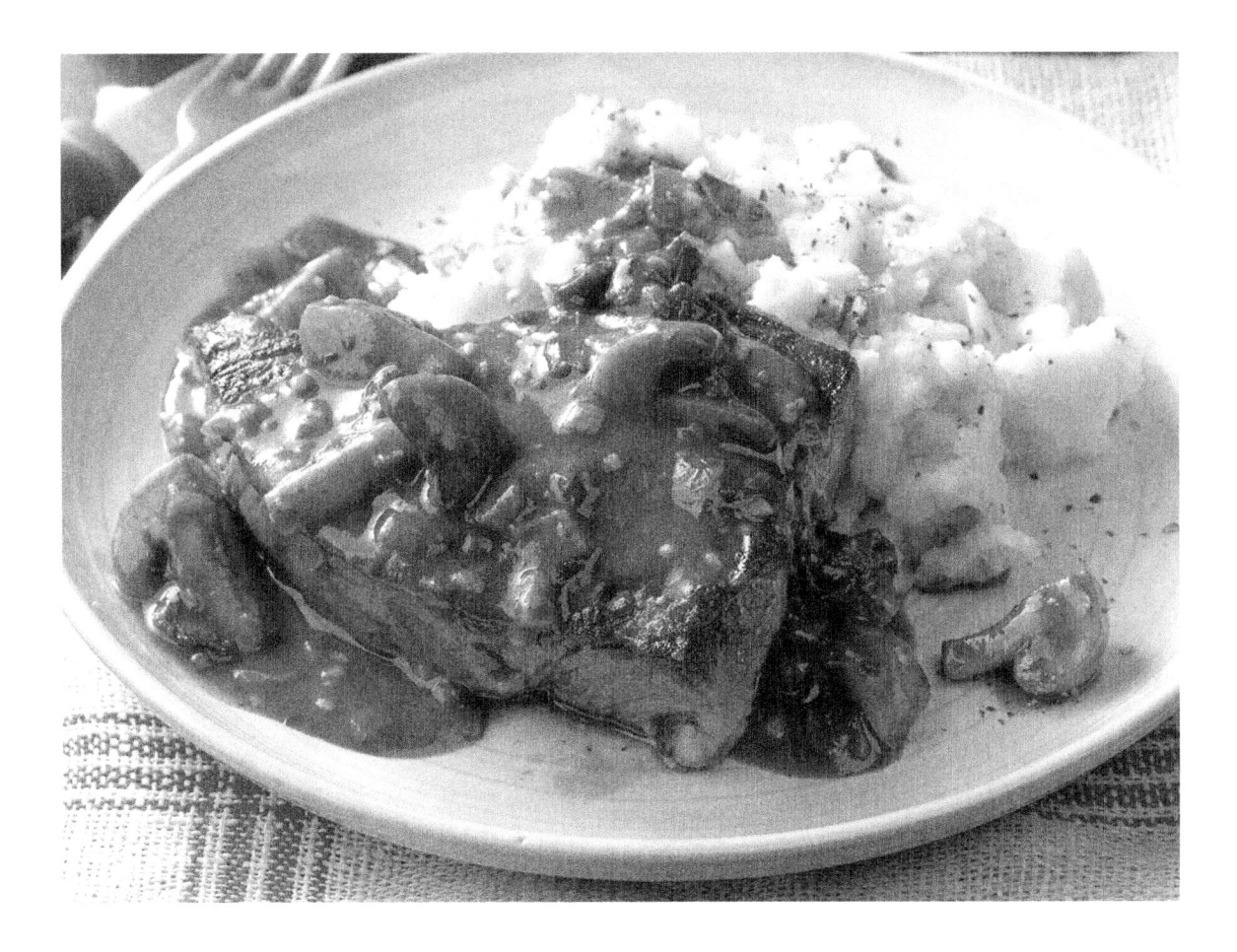

Prepare this one-skillet dinner composed of steak, peas, and broccoli rabe when you want something special but don't have the luxury of time.

Serving Size: 4

Preparation Cooking Time: 30 minutes

Ingredients:

- 12 oz. sirloin steak, fat trimmed
- 2 teaspoons grilling seasoning (unsalted)
- 2 teaspoons vegetable oil
- 6 oz. broccoli rabe, trimmed
- 2 cups peas
- 3 cups fresh mushrooms, sliced
- 1 tablespoon whole-grain mustard
- 1 cup beef broth (unsalted)
- Salt to taste
- 2 teaspoons cornstarch

Instructions:

1. Preheat your oven to 350 degrees F.

2. Sprinkle both sides of the meat with the seasoning.

3. Cook the steak and broccoli rabe in a pan over medium high heat for 4 minutes.

4. Add the peas around the steak.

5. Transfer the pan to the oven and bake for 8 minutes.

6. Transfer the beef and veggies to a plate.

7. Cook the mushrooms in the pan drippings for 3 minutes.

8. Stir in the rest of the ingredients.

9. Cook while stirring for 1 minute.

10. Pour the gravy over the steak and veggies.

Nutrients per Serving:

- Calories 226
- Fat 6.4 g
- Saturated fat 1.5 g
- Carbohydrates 16.4 g
- Fiber 5.1 g
- Protein 26.5 g
- Cholesterol 51 mg
- Sugars 6 g
- Sodium 356 mg
- Potassium 780 mg

Chicken Pasta Primavera

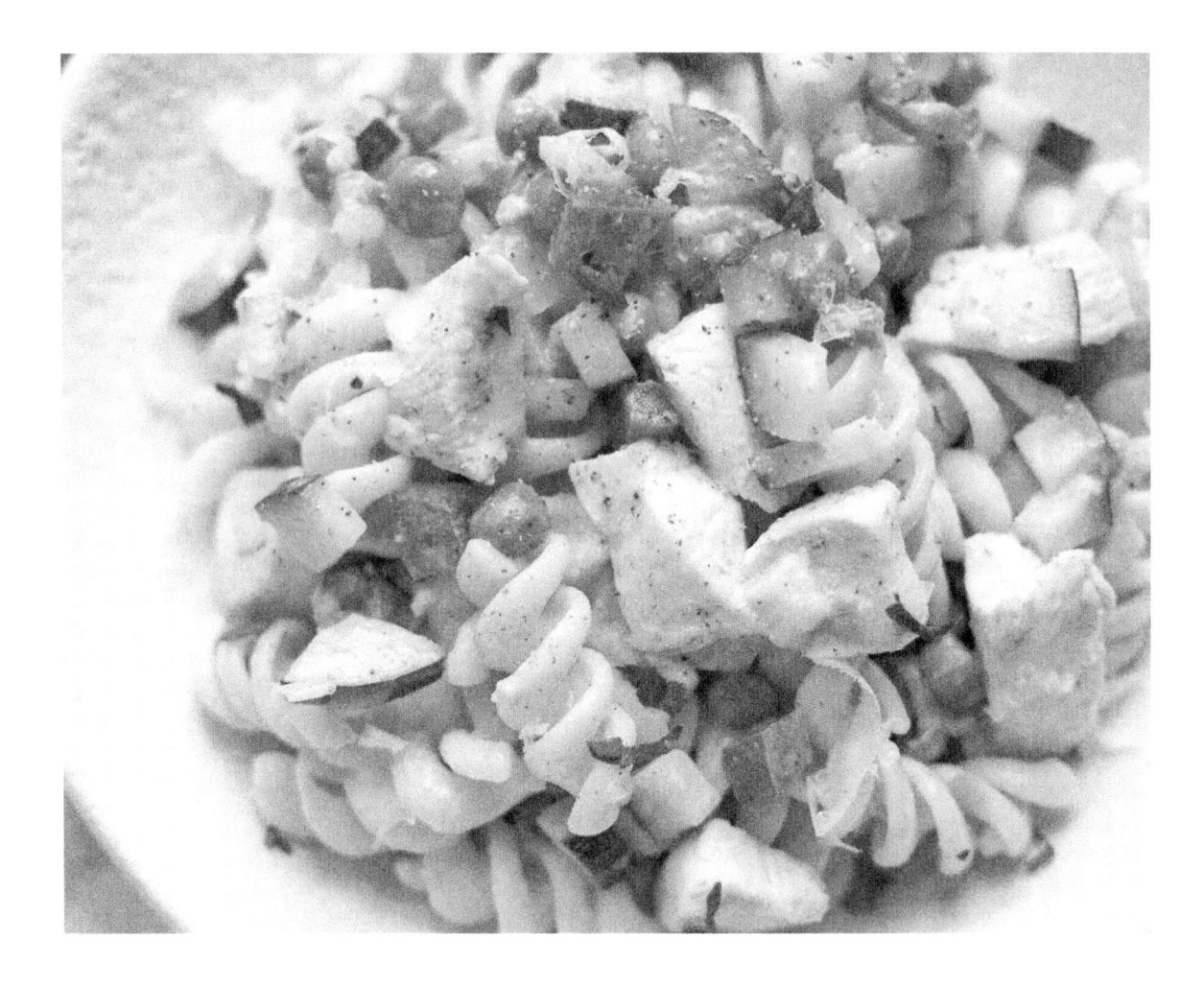

Perfect for a busy weeknight, this chicken pasta primavera requires minimal preparation but gives you outstanding results.

Serving Size: 2

Preparation Cooking Time: 50 minutes

Ingredients:

- 2 teaspoons olive oil
- ¼ cup onion, chopped
- 1 clove garlic, crushed and minced
- ½ cup low-sodium chicken broth
- 2 cups cauliflower florets
- Salt and pepper to taste
- 3 tablespoons Parmesan cheese, shredded
- ¼ cup water
- 3 oz. spaghetti
- Cooking spray
- 4 chicken breast tenderloins, sliced in half
- 2 tablespoons fresh basil leaves, snipped
- 2 cups broccoli florets, chopped and steamed
- 1 cup red sweet pepper, sliced into strips and cooked

Instructions:

1. In a pan over medium heat, cook the onion and garlic for 3 minutes.

2. Pour in the broth and add the cauliflower.

3. Bring to a boil.

4. Reduce heat and simmer for 15 minutes.

5. Transfer the mixture to a food processor.

6. Pulse until smooth.

7. Pour in the water, salt, pepper and cheese.

8. Pulse until well combined.

9. Prepare the pasta according to the directions in the package.

10. Spray your pan with oil.

11. Place it over medium heat.

12. Cook the chicken for 5 minutes per side.

13. Add the sauce and pasta.

14. Serve immediately.

Nutrients per Serving:

- Calories 451
- Fat 12.1 g
- Saturated fat 2.8 g
- Carbohydrates 44.9 g
- Fiber 8.8 g
- Protein 41.8 g
- Cholesterol 88 mg
- Sugars 9 g
- Sodium 527 mg
- Potassium 1183 mg

Lemon Chicken

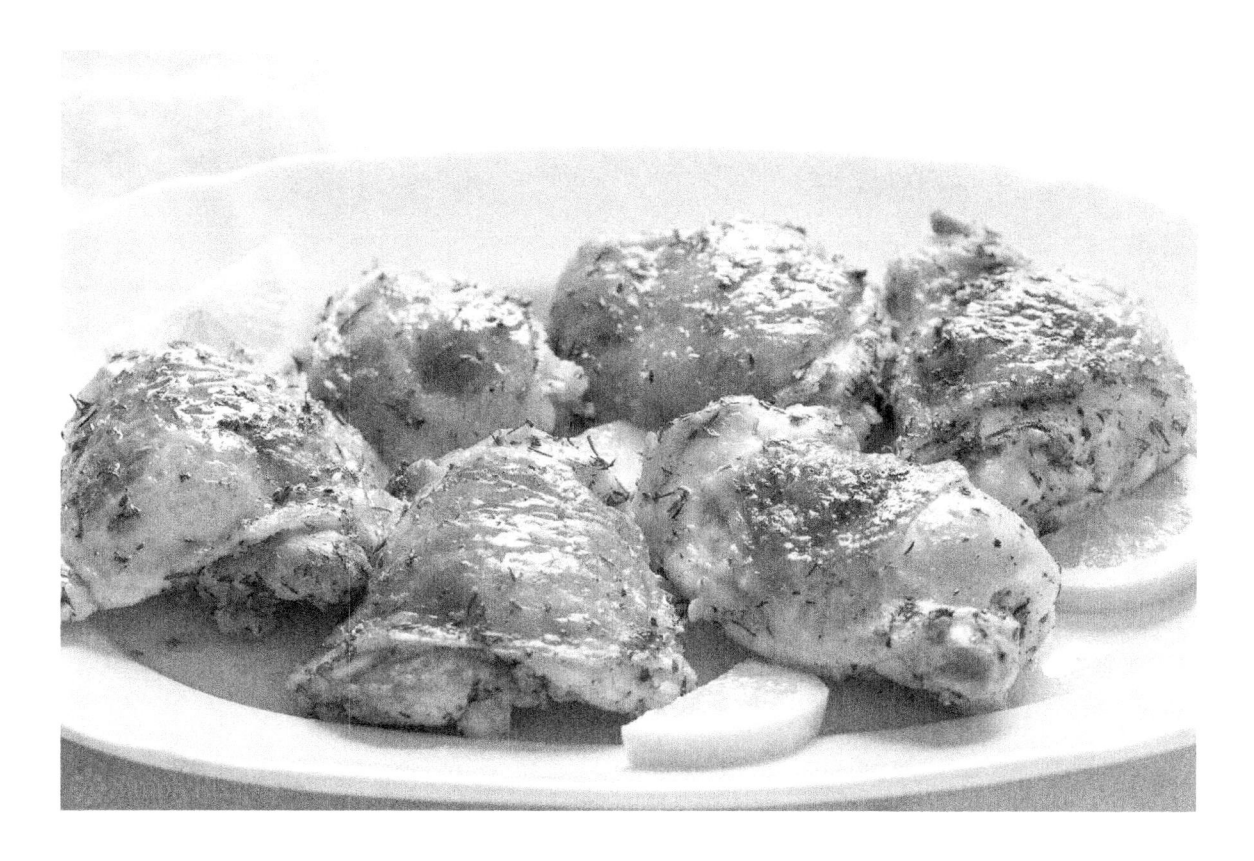

This recipe is so easy that you'd probably add this to your weekly menu. But you can expect that you won't get bored with the delicious flavors.

Serving Size: 4

Preparation Cooking Time: 1 hour and 30 minutes

Ingredients:

- ¾ cup freshly squeezed lemon juice
- 2 teaspoons lemon zest
- Salt to taste
- 1 tablespoon olive oil
- 1 teaspoon red pepper flakes
- 4 cloves garlic, crushed and minced
- 5 oz. chicken breast fillet
- 20 cherry tomatoes
- 1 lb. Brussels sprouts, trimmed and steamed

Instructions:

1. In a bowl, mix the lemon juice, lemon zest, salt, olive oil, red pepper flakes and garlic.

2. Set aside ¼ cup of this mixture.

3. Add the chicken to the remaining mixture in the bowl.

4. Cover the bowl and marinate in the refrigerator for 30 minutes.

5. Thread the cherry tomatoes and Brussels sprouts onto skewers.

6. Grill until charred.

7. Brush with the reserved sauce.

8. Grill the chicken until fully cooked.

9. Serve the chicken with the skewered veggies.

Nutrients per Serving:

- Calories 234
- Fat 5.1 g
- Saturated fat 1 g
- Carbohydrates 13.7 g
- Fiber 5 g
- Protein 34.4 g
- Cholesterol 91 mg
- Sugars 5 g
- Sodium 236 mg
- Potassium 1140 mg

Citrus Salmon Grilled Veggies

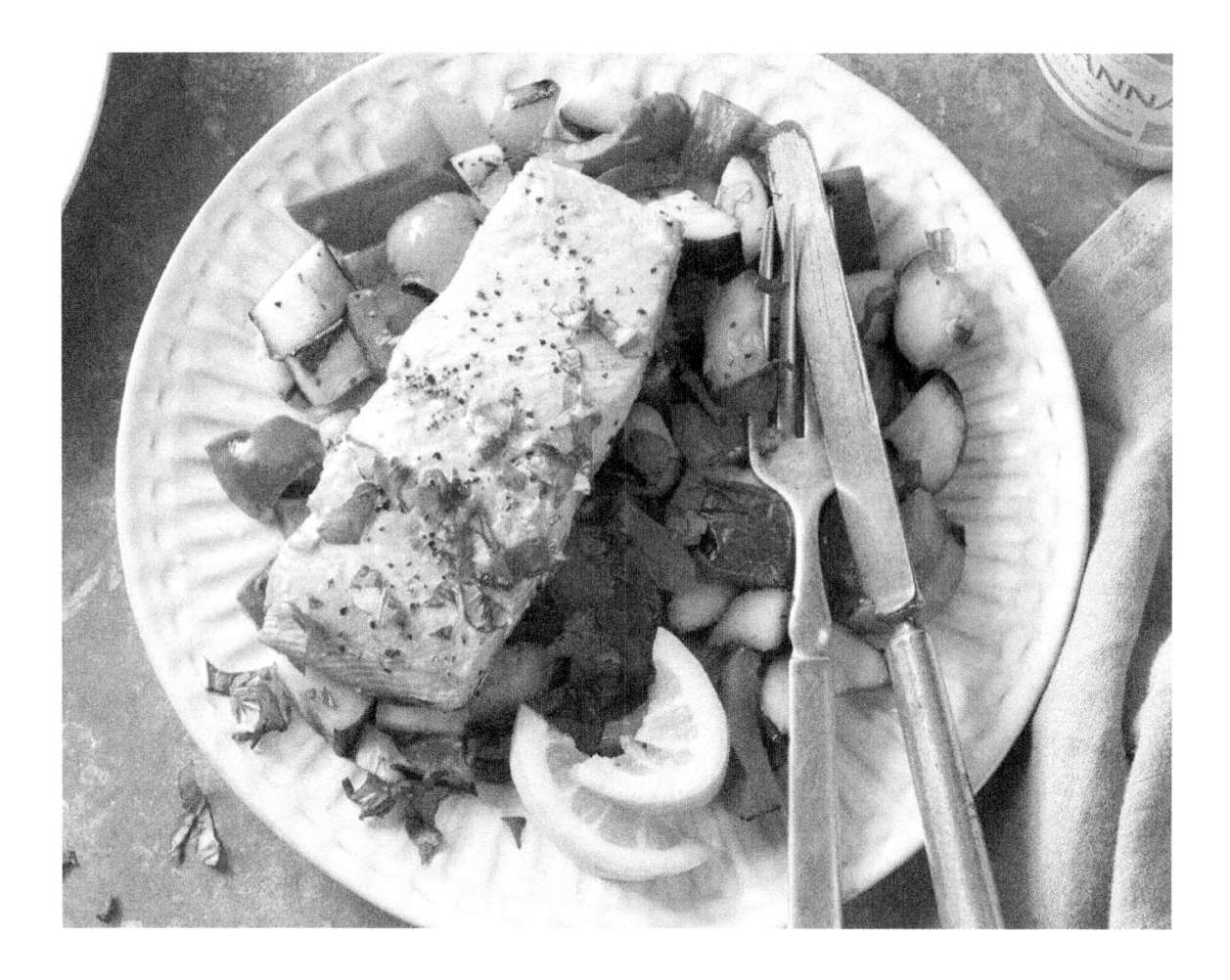

This is one of the simplest, but at the same time, this is the most delicious way to prepare salmon. The combinations of herbs and garlic transform salmon into something that you will crave for.

Serving Size: 4

Preparation Cooking Time: 1 hour and 30 minutes

Ingredients:

- ½ cup garlic and herb seasoning (unsalted)
- Salt to taste
- ¼ cup freshly squeezed orange juice
- 6 tablespoons green onions, sliced thinly and divided
- 4 salmon fillets
- Cooking spray
- 1 summer squash, sliced
- 1 lb. asparagus, sliced
- Pepper to taste
- 4 teaspoons vegetable oil
- Orange wedges or slices

Instructions:

1. Place the salmon in a dish.

2. In a bowl, combine the garlic and herb seasoning, salt, orange juice and 2 tablespoons green onion.

3. Add the salmon and turn to coat evenly.

4. Cover the bowl with foil.

5. Marinate inside the refrigerator for 1 hour.

6. Preheat your grill.

7. In a bowl, combine the squash, asparagus and remaining green onion.

8. Spray with oil.

9. Season with the pepper.

10. Make a foil packet.

11. Add the vegetables inside the foil packet and seal.

12. Add the packet on the grill and cook for 5 minutes per side.

13. Add the salmon in a skillet over medium heat.

14. Cook for 3 minutes per side.

15. Serve the salmon with the grilled veggies and orange wedges.

Nutrients per Serving:

- Calories 259
- Fat 13.9 g
- Saturated fat 1.5 g
- Carbohydrates 9.7 g
- Fiber 3.1 g
- Protein 25.7 g
- Cholesterol 62 mg
- Sugars 5 g
- Sodium 407 mg
- Potassium 947 mg

Beef Kebab

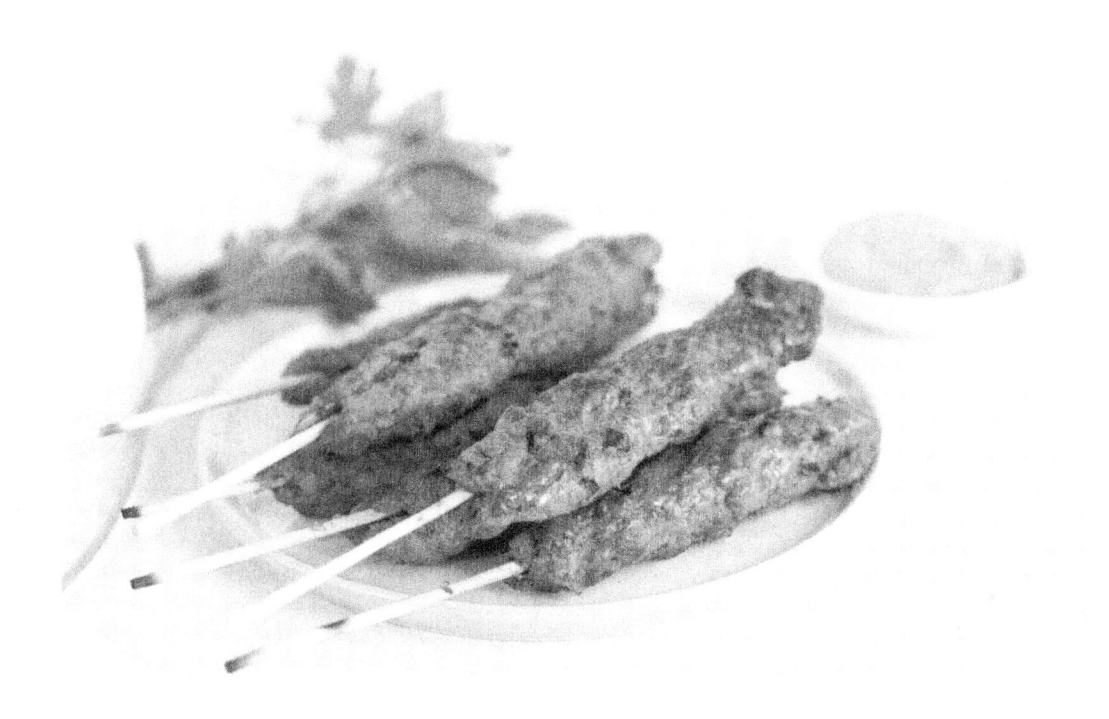

Craving for a kebab? Try this recipe that goes perfectly with chimichurri sauce.

Serving Size: 4

Preparation Cooking Time: 4 hours and 40 minutes

Ingredients:

Beef

- 1 tablespoon olive oil
- 2 cloves garlic, crushed and minced
- 1 tablespoon freshly squeezed lemon juice
- 1 teaspoon freshly grated lemon zest
- ½ teaspoon ground cumin
- 1 tablespoon fresh oregano, snipped
- Salt and pepper to taste
- 1 lb. beef sirloin steak, fat trimmed and sliced into cubes

Chimichurri

- 2 tablespoons olive oil
- 2 shallots, chopped
- 3 cloves garlic, peeled
- 2 tablespoons fresh oregano leaves
- 1 ¼ cups Italian parsley leaves
- 1 tablespoon freshly squeezed lemon juice
- 2 tablespoons cider vinegar
- ⅛ teaspoon red pepper flakes
- Salt to taste
- Vegetables
- 8 oz. small onions, peeled and boiled
- 1 green sweet pepper, sliced
- 8 oz. large button mushrooms

Instructions:

1. In a bowl, combine the olive oil, garlic, lemon juice, lemon zest, ground cumin, oregano, salt and pepper.

2. Mix well.

3. Add the beef and turn to coat evenly.

4. Cover the bowl with foil.

5. Marinate in the refrigerator for 4 hours.

6. While waiting, add all the chimichurri ingredients in the food processor.

7. Pulse until smooth.

8. Transfer to a bowl.

9. Chill in the refrigerator for 2 hours.

10. Thread the beef cubes and vegetables onto skewers.

11. Get 1 tablespoon of chimichurri and brush the kebabs with this sauce.

12. Grill the kebabs for 4 to 6 minutes per side.

13. Serve with the remaining sauce.

Nutrients per Serving:

- Calories 281
- Fat 15.9 g
- Saturated fat 3.2 g
- Carbohydrates 14 g
- Fiber 3.2 g
- Protein 23.2 g
- Cholesterol 61 mg
- Sugars 5 g
- Sodium 506 mg
- Potassium 849 mg

Grilled Veggies

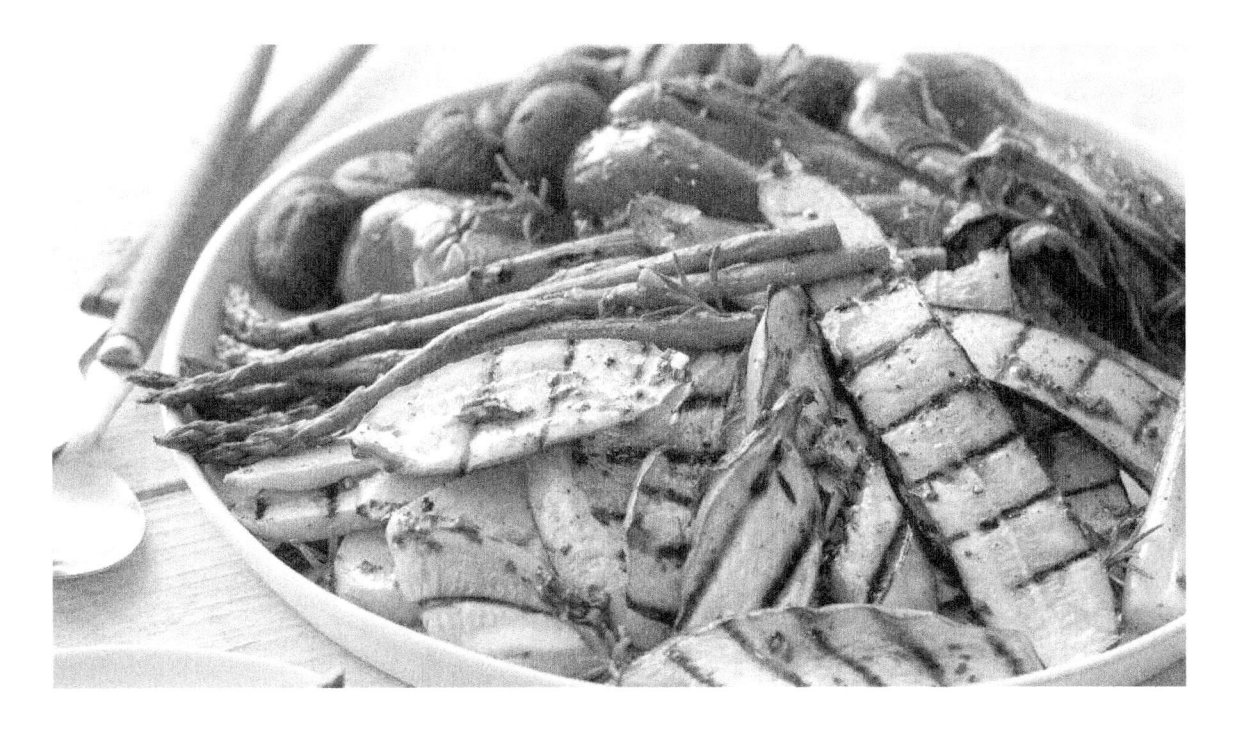

Marinate your favorite veggies in a flavorful sauce and then grill them to perfection—a perfect meal, even for busy days.

Serving Size: 6

Preparation Cooking Time: 45 minutes

Ingredients:

- 3 tablespoons olive oil
- ¼ cup balsamic vinegar
- 2 cloves garlic, crushed and minced
- 1 tablespoon fresh basil leaves, snipped
- Salt and pepper to taste
- 2 red sweet peppers, sliced into strips
- 2 yellow sweet peppers, sliced into strips
- 8 oz. fresh asparagus, trimmed and sliced
- 6 mushrooms
- 1 bulb fennel, sliced into segments
- 2 zucchinis, sliced
- 2 eggplants, sliced

Instructions:

1. In a bowl, combine the olive oil, vinegar, garlic, basil leaves, salt and pepper.

2. Toss the vegetables in the marinade.

3. Grill the vegetables until crispy but tender.

4. Arrange on a serving plate.

Nutrients per Serving:

- Calories 155
- Fat 7.4 g
- Saturated fat 1 g
- Carbohydrates 20.4 g
- Fiber 6.9 g
- Protein 4.5 g
- Cholesterol 13 mg
- Sugars 9 g
- Sodium 133 mg
- Potassium 871 mg

Garlic Fish

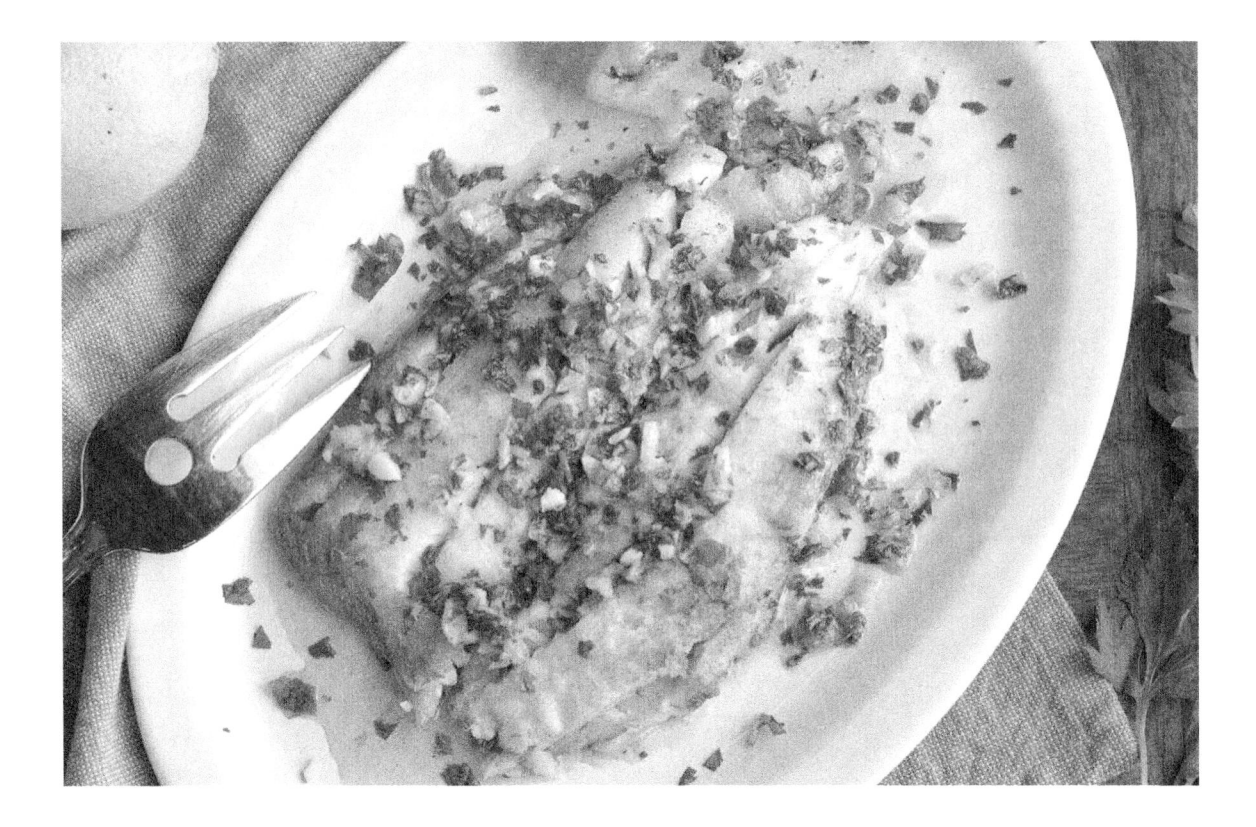

Fish marinated in creamy garlic sauce and grilled golden—this is sure to entice everyone in your family.

Serving Size: 4

Preparation Cooking Time: 2 hours and 30 minutes

Ingredients:

- ½ onion, sliced
- 6 cloves garlic, sliced
- ½ red sweet pepper, sliced
- 2 tablespoons olive oil
- ¼ cup dry white wine
- 2 teaspoons sweet paprika
- 2 tablespoons ketchup
- ¼ cup fresh cilantro, snipped
- Salt and pepper to taste
- 1 ½ lb. fish fillets

Instructions:

1. Add the onion, garlic, red sweet pepper, olive oil, white wine, sweet paprika, ketchup, cilantro, salt and pepper in a food processor.

2. Pulse until smooth.

3. Transfer half of this mixture to a bowl.

4. Cover and put inside the refrigerator.

5. Spread the remaining mixture on both sides of the fish.

6. Place on a plate.

7. Cover with foil.

8. Marinate in the refrigerator for 2 hours.

9. Grill the fish for 4 to 6 minutes per side.

10. Serve with the remaining sauce on top.

Nutrients per Serving:

- Calories 256
- Fat 6.7 g
- Saturated fat 1.1 g
- Carbohydrates 4.9 g
- Fiber 0.9 g
- Protein 40.5 g
- Cholesterol 76 mg
- Sugars 2 g
- Sodium 321 mg
- Potassium 859 mg

Mexican Chicken Salad

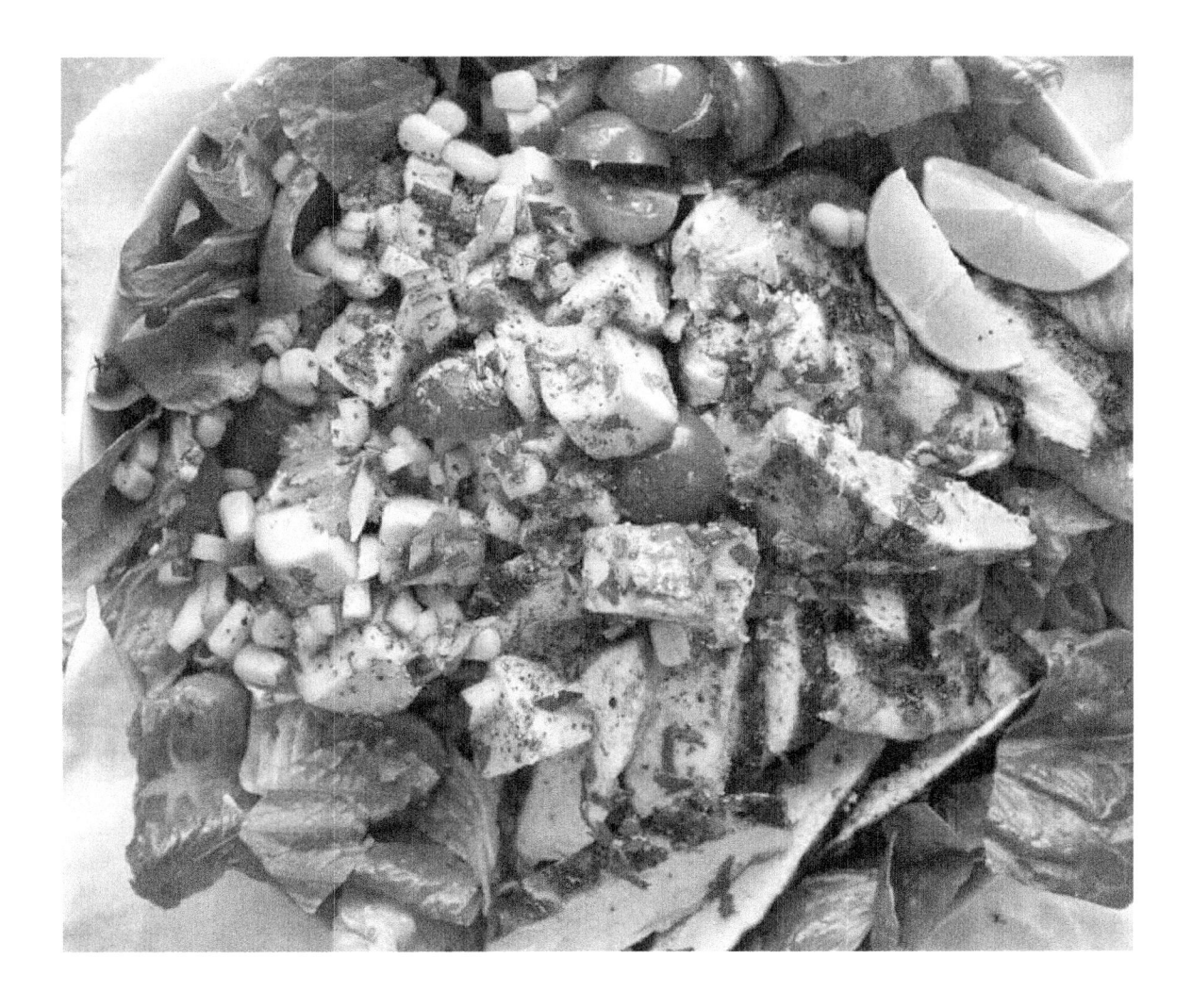

If you're looking for something different to try, opt for this Mexican-inspired chicken salad, which can be ready within a few minutes.

Serving Size: 4

Preparation Cooking Time: 40 minutes

Ingredients:

- 4 chicken breast fillets
- Salt and pepper to taste
- 1 teaspoon chili powder
- ½ teaspoon dried thyme, crushed
- ½ teaspoon dried oregano, crushed
- 1 tablespoon olive oil
- 1 teaspoon honey
- 2 tablespoons freshly squeezed orange juice
- 1 tablespoon white wine vinegar
- 4 cups Romaine lettuce, shredded
- 2 oranges, peeled and separated into sections
- 1 avocado, sliced
- ¼ cup Monterey Jack cheese, grated

Instructions:

1. Wrap the chicken breast fillet with cling wrap. Pound the chicken to flatten.

2. Preheat your broiler.

3. In a bowl, mix the salt, pepper, chili powder, thyme and oregano.

4. Sprinkle both sides with the spice mixture.

5. Broil for 4 minutes per side.

6. Slice the chicken into strips.

7. In another bowl, combine the olive oil, honey, orange juice and vinegar.

8. Stir in the lettuce.

9. Top with the chicken, oranges, avocado and cheese.

Nutrients per Serving:

- Calories 306
- Fat 13.3 g
- Saturated fat 2.7 g
- Carbohydrates 18.2 g
- Fiber 7.1 g
- Protein 30.1 g
- Cholesterol 68 mg
- Sugars 11 g
- Sodium 153 mg
- Potassium 775 mg

Nori Wrapped Fish

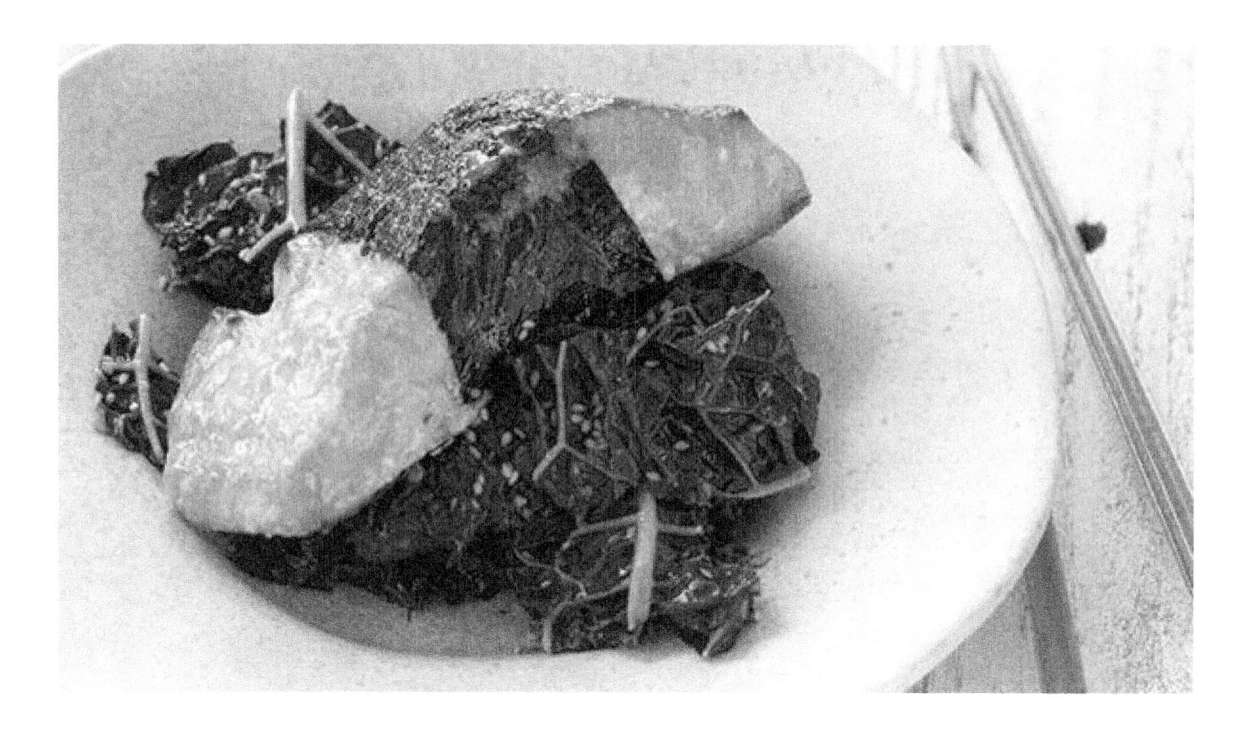

Wrap your salmon with nori and serve with beet and carrot salad for a delicious meal that you can enjoy without having to worry about your health.

Serving Size: 4

Preparation Cooking Time: 2 hours and 30 minutes

Ingredients:

- 2 carrots, sliced using a peeler
- 8 baby beets, sliced and boiled
- 2 teaspoons sugar
- 2 tablespoons rice vinegar
- Pinch ground ginger
- Salt and pepper to taste
- 4 salmon fillets
- Cooking spray
- 4 teaspoons wasabi mustard
- 4 sheets nori

Instructions:

1. Combine the carrots, beets, sugar, vinegar, ginger, salt and pepper in a bowl.

2. Cover with foil.

3. Chill in the refrigerator for 2 hours.

4. Preheat your oven to 400 degrees F.

5. Spray your baking pan with oil.

6. Spread the wasabi mustard in the middle part of the nori sheet.

7. Add the fish fillets on top of the wasabi.

8. Sprinkle with the pepper.

9. Wrap the fish.

10. Place the wrapped fish in the baking pan.

11. Bake for 15 minutes.

12. Serve with the carrot and beet mixture.

Nutrients per Serving:

- Calories 248
- Fat 4.8 g
- Saturated fat 1.1 g
- Carbohydrates 15.9 g
- Fiber 3.9 g
- Protein 35.3 g
- Cholesterol 13 mg
- Sugars 11 g
- Sodium 473 mg
- Potassium 977 mg

Roasted Acorn Squash

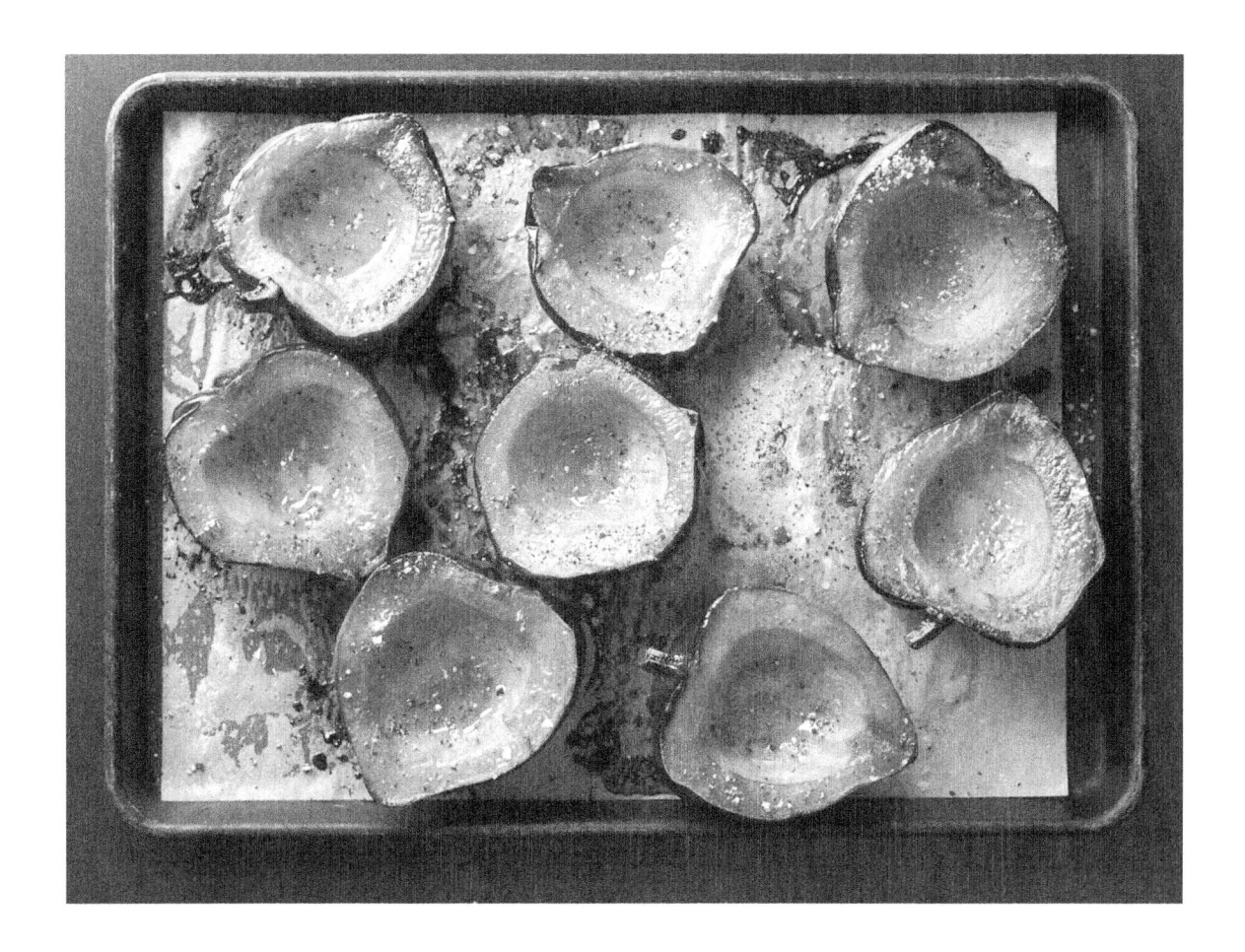

Create this simple but attractive and delicious meal for you and your whole family to enjoy. Simply roast acorn squash slices seasoned with herbs like rosemary and glazed with butter.

Serving Size: 4

Preparation Cooking Time: 1 hour and 10 minutes

Ingredients:

- 2 acorn squash, sliced
- ¾ cup low-sodium vegetable broth
- 2 cloves garlic, sliced thinly
- Salt and pepper to taste
- 2 tablespoons light butter
- 1 teaspoon fresh rosemary, snipped

Instructions:

1. Preheat your oven to 350 degrees F.

2. Pour the broth into a baking pan and add the garlic.

3. Arrange the slices of acorn squash in the baking pan.

4. Season with the salt and pepper.

5. Cover with foil.

6. Bake for 40 minutes.

7. Remove the cover and bake for another 10 minutes.

8. Transfer squash slices to a serving plate.

9. Transfer the liquid from the baking pan into a pan over medium heat.

10. Stir in the butter and rosemary.

11. Pour the butter mixture over the roasted squash and serve.

Nutrients per Serving:

- Calories 155
- Fat 3.2 g
- Saturated fat 1.8 g
- Carbohydrates 25.4 g
- Fiber 3.5 g
- Protein 2 g
- Cholesterol 8 mg
- Sugars 2 g
- Sodium 205 mg
- Potassium 826 mg

Vegetable Fruit Plate

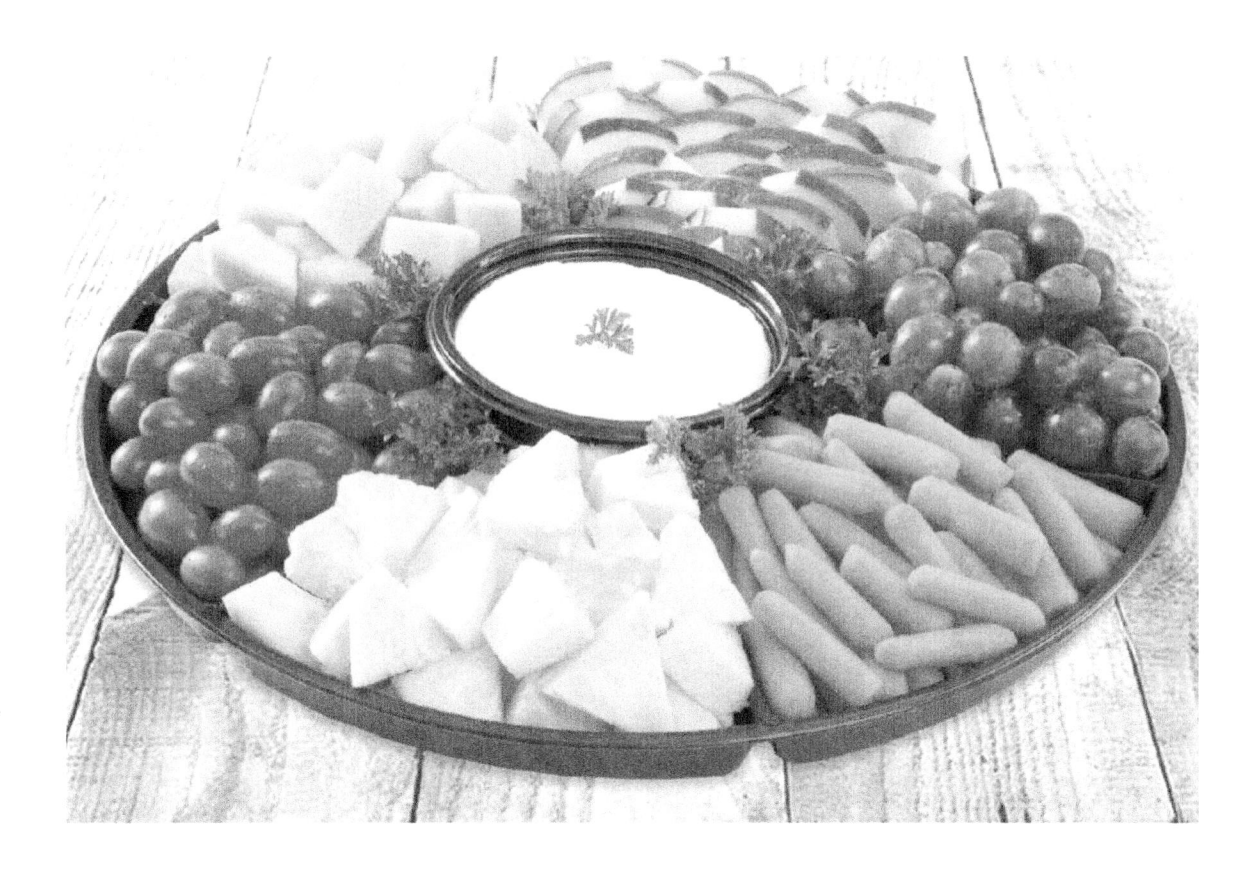

Serve fresh vegetables and sweet fruits with white bean dip. It's a quick way to serve snacks to friends coming over to your home.

Serving Size: 4

Preparation Cooking Time: 10 minutes

Ingredients:

- ¾ cup white bean dip
- 1 cup green beans, trimmed and steamed
- 8 baby bell peppers
- 20 olives
- 2 cups watermelon, sliced into cubes
- 1 cup red grapes
- 20 crackers (unsalted)
- ½ cup roasted pepitas (unsalted)

Instructions:

1. Arrange the ingredients in a serving platter and serve.

Nutrients per Serving:

- Calories 654
- Fat 30.3 g
- Saturated fat 2.9 g
- Carbohydrates 83.7 g
- Fiber 11.4 g
- Protein 13.9 g
- Cholesterol 8 mg
- Sugars 39 g
- Sodium 568 mg
- Potassium 782 mg

Herbed Fish Veggies

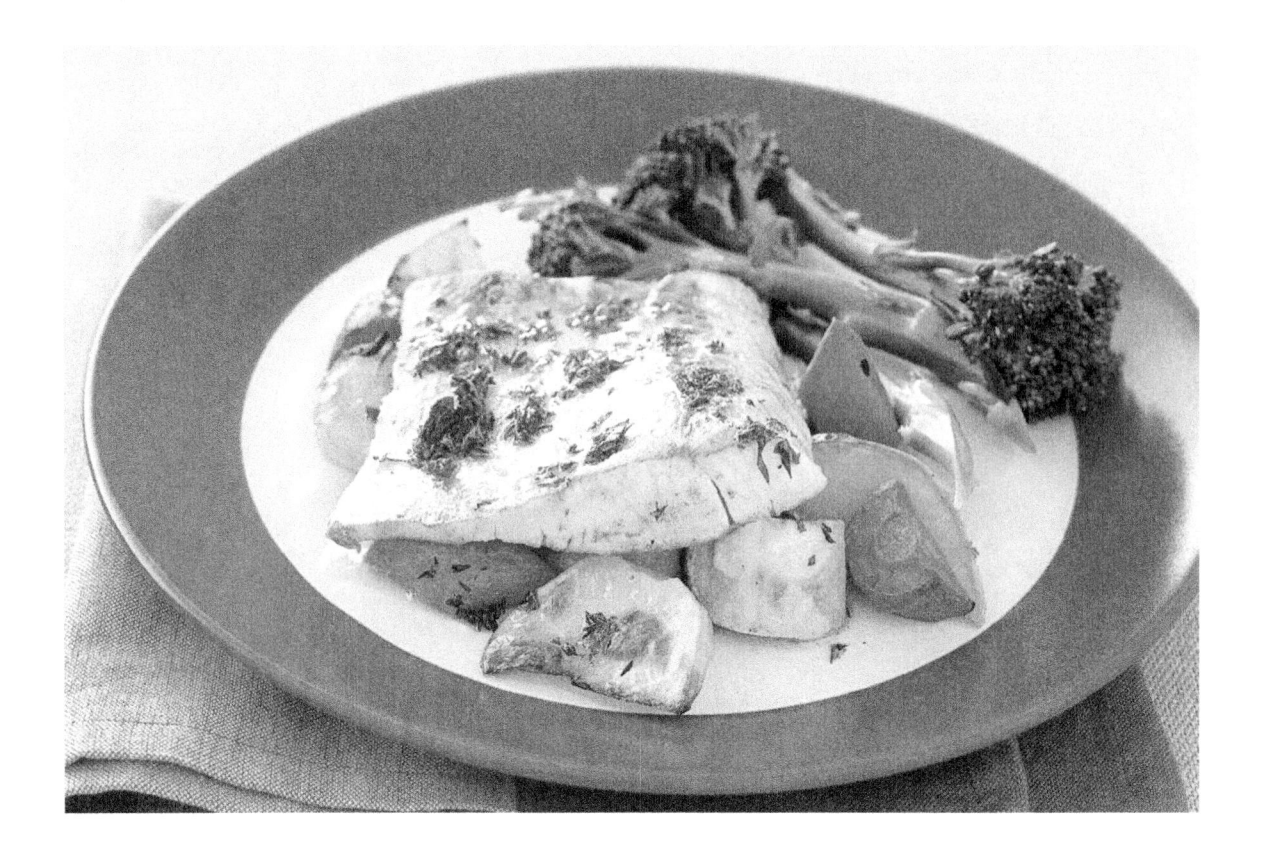

Here's a quick meal that you can prepare within 20 minutes but won't disappoint you when it comes to quality and taste.

Serving Size: 2

Preparation Cooking Time: 30 minutes

Ingredients:

- 2 cod fillets
- ½ tablespoon parsley, chopped
- ½ tablespoon oregano, chopped
- ½ tablespoon basil, chopped
- ½ tablespoon thyme, chopped
- 1 cup squash, sliced into thin strips
- 1 cup carrot, sliced into thin strips
- ½ lemon, sliced thinly
- 3 tablespoons light mayonnaise
- 1 teaspoon freshly squeezed lemon juice
- ¼ teaspoon freshly grated lemon zest
- 1 tablespoon green onion, chopped

Instructions:

1. Make shallow cuts on the fish fillets.

2. Sprinkle each with the herbs.

3. Add water to a pan.

4. Place a steamer basket inside the pan.

5. Add the squash and carrots to the steamer basket.

6. Arrange the fish on top of the veggies.

7. Top the fish with the lemon slices.

8. Cover the pan and steam for 7 minutes.

9. In a bowl, combine the rest of the ingredients.

10. Serve the fish and veggies with the mayo mixture.

Nutrients per Serving:

- Calories 270
- Fat 9.8 g
- Saturated fat 1.7 g
- Carbohydrates 13.2 g
- Fiber 3.8 g
- Protein 34 g
- Cholesterol 90 mg
- Sugars 6 g
- Sodium 340 mg
- Potassium 1039 mg

Roasted Fish with Veggies

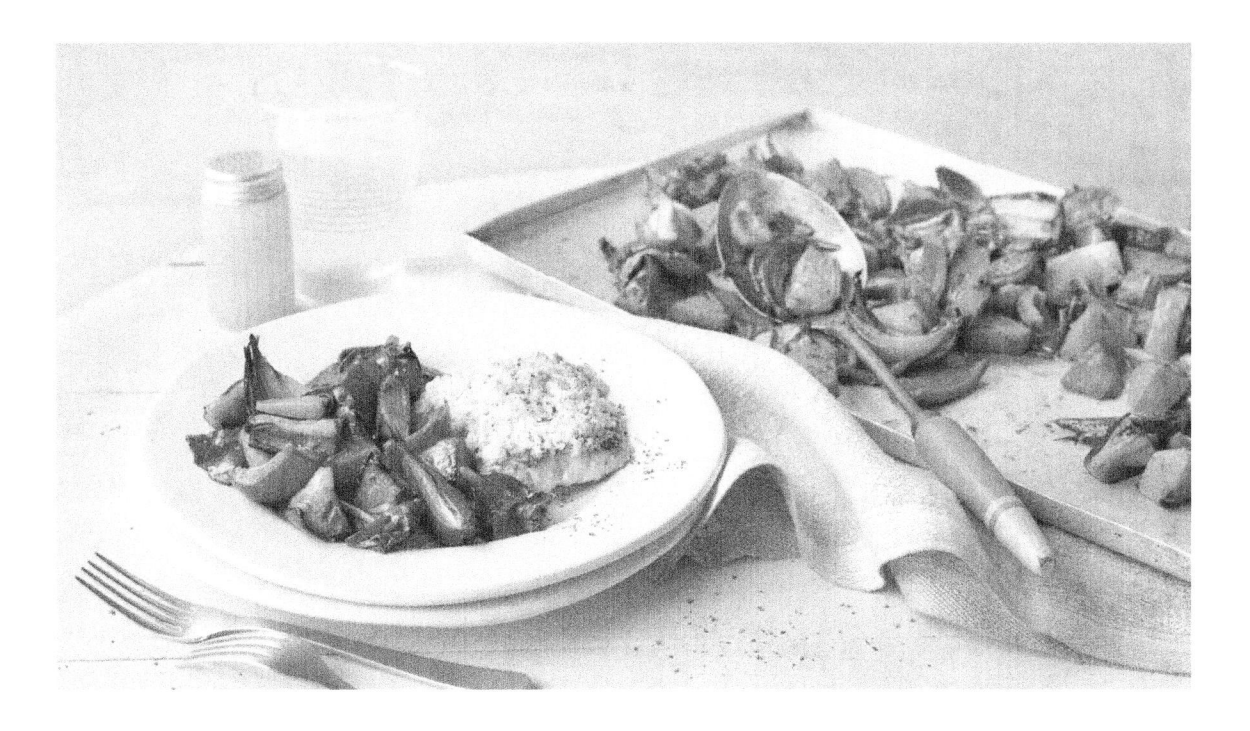

Whether you're having a family dinner at home or wondering what to bring to your next potluck, here's a recipe that won't ever fail you. It's quick, simple, but full of flavor.

Serving Size: 4

Preparation Cooking Time: 40 minutes

Ingredients:

- 4 cod fillets
- 1 onion, sliced thinly
- 1 cup button mushrooms, sliced in half
- 2 cups peas
- ¾ cup grape tomatoes
- 4 teaspoons olive oil, divided
- Salt and pepper to taste
- 2 teaspoons fresh dill, snipped

Instructions:

1. Preheat your oven to 425 degrees F.

2. Spray your baking pan with oil.

3. In a bowl, combine the onion, mushrooms, peas and tomatoes.

4. Toss in half of the oil, and season with the salt and pepper.

5. Roast in the oven for 10 minutes.

6. Push the vegetables on one side of the pan.

7. Place the fish on the other side.

8. Brush with the remaining oil and sprinkle with the salt and pepper.

9. Roast for 12 minutes.

10. Garnish with the dill before serving.

Nutrients per Serving:

- Calories 228
- Fat 5.8 g
- Saturated fat 0.9 g
- Carbohydrates 13.3 g
- Fiber 3.9 g
- Protein 30.2 g
- Cholesterol 60 mg
- Sugars 6 g
- Sodium 306 mg
- Potassium 871 mg

Salmon Veggies

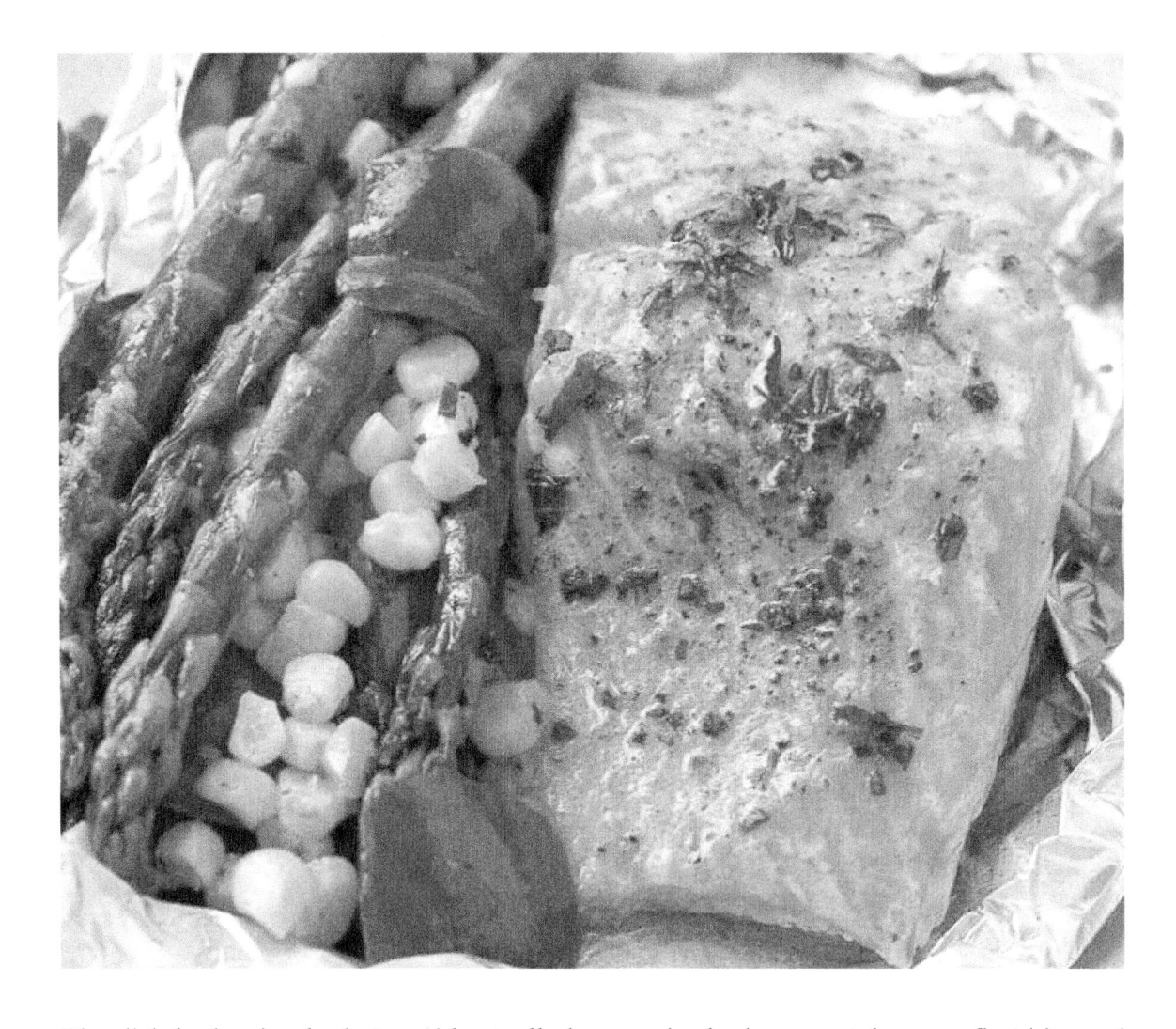

The dish looks simply, but you'd actually be surprised when you take your first bite and find out for yourself that it's rich in delicious flavors.

Serving Size: 1

Preparation Cooking Time: 30 minutes

Ingredients:

- 3 oz. salmon fillet
- ½ teaspoon dried rosemary
- ½ teaspoon dried parsley
- ½ tomato, sliced
- ½ cup asparagus spears, roasted
- ½ cup roasted red potatoes, sliced into wedges
- ¼ cup low-fat yogurt

Instructions:

1. Season the salmon with the parsley and rosemary.

2. Grill or steam until cooked and flaky.

3. Serve the fish with the vegetables and yogurt.

Nutrients per Serving:

- Calories 289
- Fat 10.6 g
- Saturated fat 1.6 g
- Carbohydrates 21.8 g
- Fiber 3.9 g
- Protein 26.7 g
- Cholesterol 60 mg
- Sugars 3 g
- Sodium 216 mg
- Potassium 918 mg

Grilled Burger

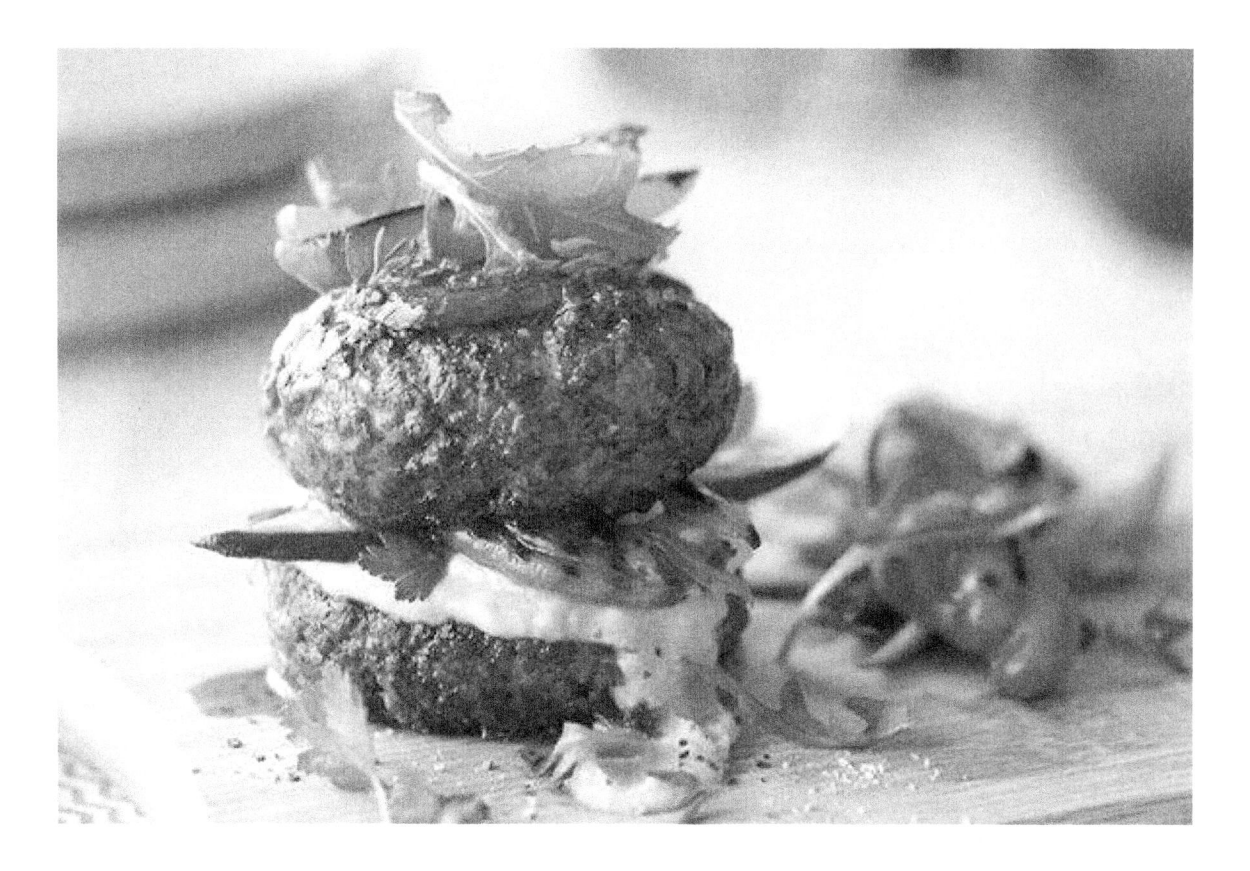

This isn't like the burger that you used to. This one is healthier as it is made with lean ground beef and served with plenty of colorful veggies.

Serving Size: 1

Preparation Cooking Time: 30 minutes

Ingredients:

- 3 oz. lean ground beef
- 1 tablespoon onion, minced
- 1 tablespoon parsley, chopped
- 1 tablespoon red bell pepper, chopped
- 1 teaspoon garlic powder
- ½ cup zucchini, sliced
- ½ cup summer squash, sliced
- ½ cup sweet potatoes, mashed

Instructions:

1. In a bowl, combine the lean ground beef, onion, parsley and red bell pepper.

2. Mix well.

3. Create patties from this mixture.

4. Preheat your grill.

5. Grill the burgers until fully cooked inside.

6. Grill the vegetable slices until grill marks appear.

7. Serve the burger with the grilled veggies and mashed sweet potatoes.

Nutrients per Serving:

- Calories 195
- Fat 4.7 g
- Saturated fat 2 g
- Carbohydrates 17.2 g
- Fiber 3.1 g
- Protein 20.8 g
- Cholesterol 53 mg
- Sugars 6 g
- Sodium 103 mg
- Potassium 842 mg

Veggie Strips with Guacamole

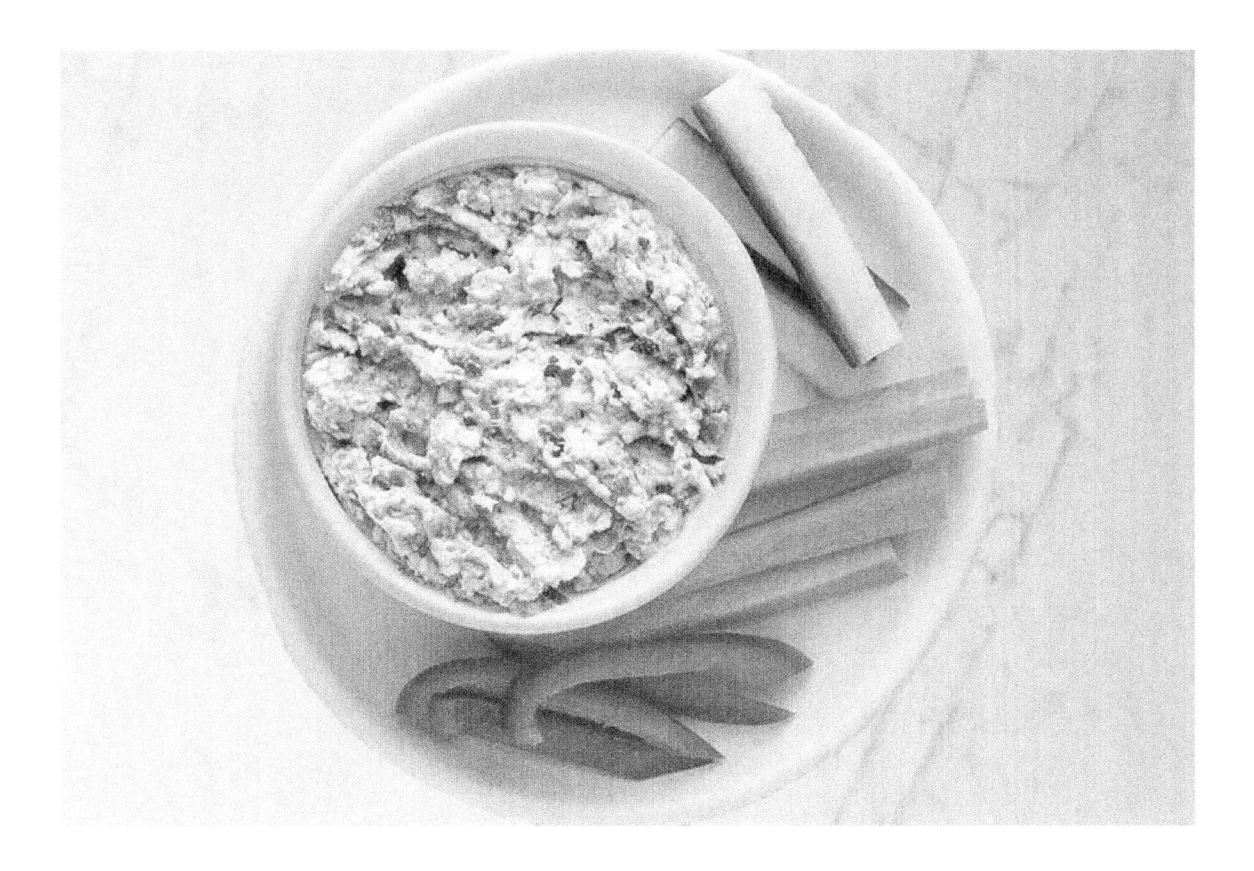

Healthy doesn't have to be bland, as proven in this quick and delicious recipe. Simply serve raw fresh veggie strips with guacamole, and it's good to go.

Serving Size: 1

Preparation Cooking Time: 5 minutes

Ingredients:

- ½ red sweet pepper, sliced into strips
- ½ yellow sweet pepper, sliced into strips
- ½ cup carrot, sliced into strips
- ¼ cup guacamole

Instructions:

1. Serve the veggie strips with the guacamole.

Nutrients per Serving:

- Calories 143
- Fat 8.3 g
- Saturated fat 1 g
- Carbohydrates 13.4 g
- Fiber 6.9 g
- Protein 3.2 g
- Cholesterol 13 mg
- Sugars 5 g
- Sodium 194 mg
- Potassium 701 mg

Conclusion

Since high blood pressure can exist with no symptoms, it's important to be vigilant.

Don't wait until you are already suffering from complications of high blood pressure. Do something about your health, your lifestyle, and your diet.

Follow the recipes in this book to create dishes that are not only healthy but also delicious and simple to prepare.

Start living healthier today.

Have a good day!

About the Author

A native of Albuquerque, New Mexico, Sophia Freeman found her calling in the culinary arts when she enrolled at the Sante Fe School of Cooking. Freeman decided to take a year after graduation and travel around Europe, sampling the cuisine from small bistros and family owned restaurants from Italy to Portugal. Her bubbly personality and inquisitive nature made her popular with the locals in the villages and when she finished her trip and came home, she had made friends for life in the places she had visited. She also came home with a deeper understanding of European cuisine.

Freeman went to work at one of Albuquerque's 5-star restaurants as a sous-chef and soon worked her way up to head chef. The restaurant began to feature Freeman's original dishes as specials on the menu and soon after, she began to write e-books with her recipes. Sophia's dishes mix local flavours with European inspiration making them irresistible to the diners in her restaurant and the online community.

Freeman's experience in Europe didn't just teach her new ways of cooking, but also unique methods of presentation. Using rich sauces, crisp vegetables and meat cooked to perfection, she creates a stunning display as well as a delectable dish. She has won many local awards for her cuisine and she continues to delight her diners with her culinary masterpieces.

Author's Afterthoughts

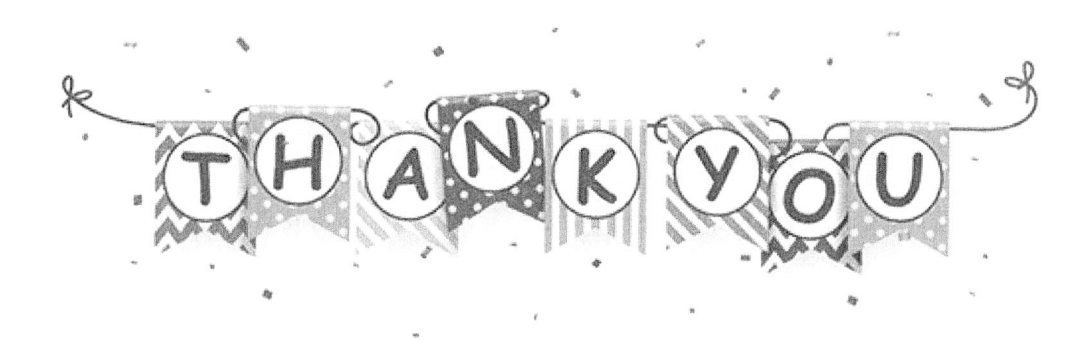

I want to convey my big thanks to all of my readers who have taken the time to read my book. Readers like you make my work so rewarding and I cherish each and every one of you.

Grateful cannot describe how I feel when I know that someone has chosen my work over all of the choices available online. I hope you enjoyed the book as much as I enjoyed writing it.

Feedback from my readers is how I grow and learn as a chef and an author. Please take the time to let me know your thoughts by leaving a review on Amazon so I and your fellow readers can learn from your experience.

My deepest thanks,

Sophia Freeman

Subscribe to the Newsletter!

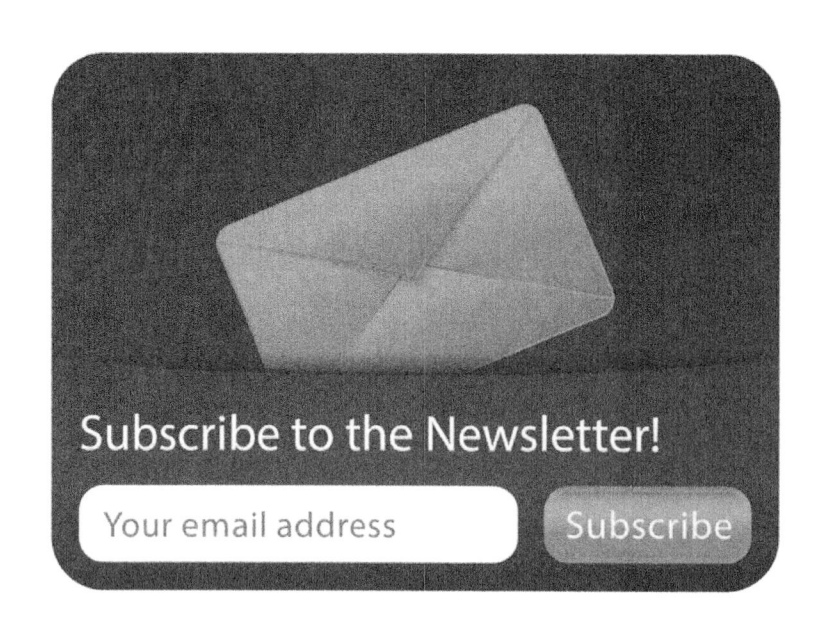

https://sophia.subscribemenow.com/

* * ★ ★ ★ ★ ★ ★ * * *

Printed in Great Britain
by Amazon